Alcohol Interventions

Historical and Sociocultural Approaches

About the Editors

David L. Strug is a Research Associate at the Hispanic Research Center of Fordham University where he is developing a program of research activities concerning alcoholism among New York State's Hispanic population. Dr. Strug's publications on alcohol and drug use are based on his ethnographic research in New York City. He has also carried out anthropological field work in Bolivia, Mexico, and Peru.

S. Priyadarsini received her Ph.D. in sociology from Rutgers University. She was a post-doctoral fellow at the Center of Alcohol Studies at Rutgers University for two years. She has carried out extensive research on crime and delinquency, and is the co-author of *Delinquency in India: A Comparative Analysis*. She has published articles on alcohol and criminal justice in a number of professional journals. Dr. Priyadarsini has taught sociology at universities both in the United States and India. She is presently the owner and President of The Village Traveler, Inc., in New York City.

Merton M. Hyman is a sociologist at the Center of Alcohol Studies, Rutgers University. His research has included studies of traffic accidents, arrests for drunk driving, follow-up studies of treated alcoholics and of state alcohol beverage control laws and practices. He editorially reviews papers on alcohol use and alcohol problems for the *Journal of Studies on Alcohol*.

Alcohol Interventions

Historical and Sociocultural Approaches

David L. Strug, S. Priyadarsini
and Merton M. Hyman
Editors

The Haworth Press
New York • London

Alcohol Interventions: Historical and Sociocultural Approaches is a monographic supplement to the journal *Alcoholism Treatment Quarterly,* Volume 2, 1985. It is not supplied as part of the subscription to the journal, but is available from the publisher at an additional charge.

Alcoholism Treatment Quarterly is the practitioner's quarterly dedicated to the needs of clinicians who work with alcoholic clients and their families.

The Haworth Press, Inc., 28 East 22 Street, New York, New York 10010-6194
EUROSPAN/Haworth, 3 Henrietta Street, London WC2E 8LU England

Library of Congress Cataloging-in-Publication Data
Main entry under title:

Alcohol interventions.

"Supplement to the journal Alcoholism treatment quarterly, volume 2, 1985"—T.p. verso.
Includes bibliographies and index.
1. Alcoholics—Rehabilitation—United States—Addresses, essays, lectures.
2. Alcoholism—Treatment—United States—History—Addresses, essays, lectures.
3. Alcoholism counseling—United States—Addresses, essays, lectures. I. Strug, David L.
II. Priyadarsini, S., 1943- . III. Hyman, Merton M. IV. Alcoholism treatment quarterly. V. 2 (Supplement) [DNLM: 1. Alcoholism—history. 2. Alcoholism—rehabilitation. W1 AL 3147 v.2 Suppl. / WM 11.1 A354]
HV5279.A69   1986   362.2'928'0973   85-16405
ISBN 0-86656-359-8
ISBN 0-86656-426-8 (pbk.)

CONTENTS

Introduction

David L. Strug
S. Priyadarsini
Merton M. Hyman

Attitudes toward alcohol use and ways of treating the heavy drinker in America have evolved over time. To understand the practices and techniques of contemporary alcohol intervention programs, it is important to have some idea of the different social contexts and social meanings that have historically been attached to alcohol use and cures for problem drinking or alcoholism. Here we use the term "alcoholism" to refer to the negative physical, psychological, and social consequences of alcohol use.

ALCOHOL USE AND SOCIOCULTURAL REACTIONS: A BRIEF OVERVIEW

What the American colonists considered "normal" drinking would be defined as deviant and intemperate from a contemporary viewpoint. Moreover, the colonists' views toward alcoholics were reflective of their basic philosophic assumptions regarding "free will" and "moral depravity" of human beings and of their class bias. Levine (1978) notes that between 1785 and 1835 the "liquor problem" became of interest to an economic and social elite increasingly concerned with drinking by the poor. The various solutions proposed by the clergy, civil authorities, and prominent persons during this time were targeted toward people of the lower social strata—the workers, farm hands, and others (Schneider, 1978).

It was also at the beginning of the late eighteenth-century—when the medical profession began to regard liquor as chemically toxic, morally destructive, and physically addictive—that the modern-day "disease concept" of alcoholism had its origin. Dr. Benjamin Rush, the well-known Philadelphia physician, was a particularly prominent spokesperson for these ideas (Keller, this volume).

The idea that alcoholism is a "disease" requiring a multifaceted treatment approach rather than a single remedy, evolved during this period. Rush stated that drunkenness "resembles certain hereditary, family and contagious diseases" (Keller, this volume). He advocated three types of measures to treat the disease: religious, metaphysical (psychological) and medical. However, Rush also administered aversion techniques to his patients. Levine (1978) points out that Rush's ideas reflected the new intellectual and philosophic developments of the age: The decline of the notion of "free will" and the recognition that one's will and desire were distinct and different.

Although Dr. Rush's experiments with behavioral and psychological treatments for alcoholism date from the eighteenth-century, the nineteenth-century witnessed the beginning of a more scientific approach to medical practice in general and medical practitioners' increasing interest in alcoholism and its treatment (Conrad and Schneider, 1980). The treatment of alcoholism fell increasingly into the province of a newly developing specialty—psychiatry. Alcoholics were treated in asylums for the inebriates. By the 1900s there were about 50 such institutions catering to the needs of alcoholics (Schneider, 1978). Thus, the idea of institutionalization and systematic treatment by professionals evolved over several decades.

The burgeoning medical science literature during the nineteenth-century in the United States invariably affected the ideas of the general culture and is reflected in the advocacy of aversion and specific aversion techniques as the remedy for alcoholism. Mass media advertisements also mirrored the widely held beliefs, myths, and ideas regarding alcohol, its impact, and its antidotes. Twentieth-century developments, such as Keeley's gold-dust treatment, reflect the ideology of this century. New scientific developments (Pavlovian conditioning and other behavioristic approaches) resulted in the administration of substances to induce vomiting when alcohol was drunk. This is still the basis of one type of contemporary treatment practice—giving Antabuse to alcoholics at the detox stage. Underlying this approach is the assumption that the unpleasantness associated with drinking while on Antabuse will deter the alcoholic from drinking any alcohol. Keller (this volume) remarks that in the 1940s the issue in the field of alcoholism treatment became whether this weaning from alcohol should be gradual or sudden, rather than the appropriateness of abstinence as a cure for alcoholism.

According to Levine (1978), in nineteenth century America, a temperance movement that "demonized" alcohol became an important social force and a rallying point for the expanding urban middle class (see also Gusfield, 1966). Thus, the liquor problem became a focus of attention for a broader sector of American society. However, this antiliquor movement evolved from temperance to Prohibition in three stages: at the beginning, only immoderate drinking was condemned; then, consuming beer and wine was defined as acceptable, but hard liquor was frowned upon; lastly, even imbibing wine and beer became repugnant.

Women played an important role in the temperance movement. Temperance leaders such as Frances Willard, Susan B. Anthony, and Carry Nation believed alcohol to be a threat to domestic life and to social status in general. A drunken husband was seen as a threat to the economic and social security of the family. Their common cause became "home protection" and was adopted as the official motto of the Woman's Christian Temperance Union (Lender, this volume).

The nineteenth century was a period of extensive social, political, and religious activism, and there were many programs for self-help and reform of the chronic drunkard. These programs were the forerunners of most contemporary treatment as well as prevention efforts. Physicians ran homes for inebriates and a number of self-help groups such as the Washingtonians, Sons of Temperance, and Good Templars came into existence (Levine, 1984). The Quarterly Journal of Inebriety began publication. Increasingly, alcohol was being perceived as "the cause" of various social ills, including poverty. Alcohol was blamed for antisocial behavior on the part of the poor and immigrants, among whom the various consequences of heavy drinking were becoming conspicuous in the industrial, urban centers of America. The leadership and financial support for the antiliquor movement came from the industrially and agriculturally wealthy, and the merchants/businessmen of the time (Levine, 1978). Keller (this volume) notes that "the very growth of treatment for alcoholics . . . was ammunition in the armory of the organized anti-liquor movement."

Underlying the temperance movement were issues such as reducing crime and poverty and defending women and children. But in the twentieth-century the rationale for dealing with drunkenness was an attack on the power of the liquor industry and the saloon—a symbol of urban, immigrant, working-class subculture (Levine, 1978). A sober, abstaining workforce meant efficiency and productivity for

American industry. Thus, diverse social segments had an interest in promoting Prohibition which came to fruition during the years between 1919 and 1933. Underlying all this activism was the fundamental assumption that alcoholism was a "social problem" to be dealt with at the societal level by means of national Prohibition (the Eighteenth Amendment).

The Reverend Harry Emerson Fosdick (cited in Levine, 1984) noted about Prohibition that: "One of the basic facts necessary to understand the prohibitory campaign is that American business found it impossible to run modern machines with drinking-befuddled brains. Canny, shrewd businesslike America knew that it would be a good financial 'bargain.' "

There were several immediate consequences of Prohibition:

> At first there was a reduction in the public manifestations of alcoholism. There were fewer arrests for drunkenness, and fewer alcoholic admissions to hospitals. The specialized alcoholism hospitals closed up, went out of business. Doctors stopped seeing alcoholic diseases. The legislative solution seemed to work and treatment of alcoholism could become an obsolete art . . . . The trouble was that it didn't work for very long. (Keller, this volume.)

However, prohibition did, apparently, have an important impact on consumption—there was a drop in the per capita alcohol consumption among the middle class (Levine, 1984).

It has been suggested that Repeal of Prohibition in 1933 (the Twenty-first Amendment) was the result not so much of an indignant America deprived of legitimate sources of alcohol, but of a number of powerful corporate interests, represented by the Association Against the Prohibition Amendment, who perceived that the restoration of liquor taxes would translate into lower personal and business taxes (Levine, 1984). Moreover, at a time of mounting social and economic pressures and protests due to the Great Depression, popular antipathy to Prohibition was also viewed as another aspect of disrespect for law and order.

Once Repeal was enacted, the windfall from taxes on alcoholic beverages was used to fund depression-relief projects (Lender and Martin, 1982). But the media images of the 1930s depicted alcohol as an integral part of the fashionable life, and associated it with the concept of masculinity (Clark, 1976).

It was during the 1930s that a stockbroker (William Wilson/Bill W.) and a doctor (Robert Holbrook Smith/Dr. Bob) got together and with financial help from the Rockefellers founded Alcoholics Anonymous (AA) (Levine, 1984). The philosophy behind this voluntary organization is that alcoholics experience loss of control over their drinking and have a progressive disease whose symptom is compulsive drinking, and the only cure is lifelong abstinence. As individuals, alcoholics are viewed as unable to control their drinking; but belonging to a group of other alcoholics, AA, helps sustain their abstinence.

Levine (1984) notes that many of these ideas date back to the temperance era; however, the major focus shifted from the danger of the substance per se to the behavior of the individual. Now alcoholism became a personal-individual problem; instead of nationwide legislation, the solution was considered to be within the realm of mutual self-help. The alcoholic seeking self-help was to be integrated into the network of "recovered alcoholics." As a consequence, the ideas of those involved in treatment for alcoholism came to be affected by those of the recovered alcoholics around them.

In addition to AA, a growing number of educational, medical, and research organizations also began to evolve around the problem of alcoholism. For example, Yale University ran several alcoholism treatment clinics. Keller (this volume) notes that in 1945 Yale University founded the first outpatient clinic to specialize in the treatment of alcoholism. A variety of treatment methods were used on patients with the hope that one or another would be compatible for some of the patients. The Yale group eagerly collaborated with AA. An important feature of the treatment program was the introduction of group therapy as a scientific tool. These original Yale clinics became models for outpatient alcoholism treatment units throughout the country.

With the growth of treatment programs and scientific interest in alcoholism, an increasing number of research reports on alcoholism began to appear in scientific and medical journals. The Research Council on Problems of Alcohol, started in 1938, further stimulated the work at Yale University. In 1939 the Council received a grant of $25,000 from the Carnegie Corporation to review the biological literature on alcohol. Dr. E. M. Jellinek was hired as project director and offices were set up in the New York Academy of Medicine. Jellinek was invited to join the Yale Center of Alcohol Studies (CAS) when it was founded in the late 1930s. The first issue of the

Quarterly Journal of Studies on Alcohol appeared in 1940. In 1943 the Summer School of Alcohol Studies (SSAS) at the Yale CAS began to train personnel involved in alcoholism treatment programs about various aspects of alcoholism (Milgram, this volume). The SSAS thus helped propagate the disease concept of alcoholism pioneered by its director, Jellinek.

In 1944 the U.S. Public Health Service labeled alcoholism the nation's fourth largest public health problem. A federal agency, thus, came to define alcoholism as a social and cultural issue. The National Committee for Education on Alcoholism was founded in the same year by Mrs. Marty Mann (an alumna of the SSAS) with the help and sponsorship of the CAS. The goal of this Committee was "to bring to all America the message that alcoholism is an illness which can be banished by therapeutic means" (Milgram, this volume). In the early 1950s this Committee changed its name to the National Council on Alcoholism (NCA) and organized large numbers of local, voluntary organizations on alcoholism across the United States.

Simultaneously, as Milgram (this volume) notes, from 1943 to 1950 there was a steady decline in the number of clergy and temperance workers who participated in the SSAS, while the number of students with professional background, such as educators, psychologists, and rehabilitation specialists, increased. The extent to which the field of alcoholism treatment was increasingly becoming professionalized can be seen in the changing curricula and the student body passing through the Yale, and later Rutgers, SSAS (Milgram, this volume).

The SSAS, now located at Rutgers University, continued to attract a large number of individuals from business, industrial, and labor groups as well as social workers and nursing professionals. The increasingly diverse student body also paralleled the increasing level of student sophistication indicated by the proportion of students with graduate training. In turn, this required that both the makeup and level of specialization of the courses offered kept pace with the changes.

In the 1950s both the American Medical Association and the American Hospital Association officially accepted and endorsed the modern disease concept of alcoholism pioneered by Jellinek, who made alcohol studies and the treatment of alcoholism respectable and legitimate by articulating them in scientific terms in *The Disease Concept of Alcoholism,* published in 1960. This study, funded by the

Christopher D. Smithers Foundation, surveyed attitudes toward the definition of alcoholism as a disease throughout the world. Two more important developments occurred during the decade between 1950 and 1960. Al-Anon was created as was the North Conway Institute. The latter was to encourage church groups to develop active ministries for alcoholics.

The evolution of the changes over 25 years in attitudes toward and the treatment of alcoholism is clearly demonstrated by a case study of alcoholism treatment in New York State (Blume, this volume). According to Blume, before 1950 the attitudes of medical professionals were uniformly negative and/or condescending; alcoholic patients were stigmatized, and in New York State there were no medical and social services for alcoholics. The 1950 Republican State Convention platform recognized alcoholism as a disease and a public-health problem requiring the development of a program of control. This plank became an administrative law in 1952. Consequently, a number of experimental outpatient programs were developed during the 1950s.

The Cooperative Commission on the Study of Alcoholism was established in 1961 with funds from the National Institute of Mental Health (NIMH). In 1967 the Commission published *Alcohol Problems: A Report to the Nation.* This Report became the basis for various federal and local activities related to alcoholism, public discussions regarding alcohol use, training programs, and research.

The 1960s and 1970s witnessed the development of a modern alcoholism constitutency and of alcohol interest and lobby groups—reflecting the nationwide boom in all kinds of activism. The Highway Safety Act of 1966 called for reports to the Congress concerning the effects of alcohol on traffic accidents. And the same year, NIMH set up a National Center for the Prevention and Control of Alcoholism under the directorship of the alcohol researcher, Jack Mendelson (Weiner, 1981).

In 1970 the Comprehensive Alcohol Abuse and Alcoholism Prevention, Treatment, and Rehabilitation Act created the National Institute on Alcohol Abuse and Alcoholism (NIAAA). This new unit gave the alcoholism constituency a seemingly permanent voice in public policy and public-health programs. For demonstration purposes, the Uniform Alcoholism and Intoxication Act of 1971 removed many alcohol-related legal infractions from the criminal-justice system, substituting medical treatment for punishment (Lender and Martin, 1982).

ABSTRACT OF ARTICLES

The articles discussed in the following sections focus on the historical and sociocultural contexts of alcoholism treatment.

Historical Developments

The premise that an individual can have control over the act of drinking is essential and basic to various self-help movements like AA. However, the act of drinking alcoholic beverages has had various shared symbolic meanings from ancient times—defined within the parameters of time, the society, and the culture. One cannot deny the fact that an alcoholic does not exist entirely in a psychological, social, and cultural vacuum. Therefore, any analysis of alcoholism treatment should pay attention to the context in which alcoholism treatment takes place—the setting, the staff, the patients, and the processes of their interaction. The following abstracts from the first four articles in this volume demonstrate a link between the various social structural dimensions of alcoholism treatment programs and ideas and beliefs concerning alcoholism and its treatment.

Mark Keller's definition of alcoholism is basic and widely accepted and distinguishes between intoxication and alcoholism (Keller, this volume). By definition, therefore, alcoholism treatment is for those with a diagnosable, addictive disease and not for the occasionally intoxicated person who is not addicted to alcohol. However, subscribing to the disease concept of alcoholism, Keller feels that many of the people who get drunk and get into trouble may be in the process of "acquiring the disease." Thus, he feels that it is necessary to learn to intervene in that process and prevent its completion.

In addressing important issues about the definition of alcoholism, Keller discusses the history of alcoholism treatment and focuses on ideas and beliefs regarding alcohol, the alcoholic, and alcoholism in their historic and cultural contexts. Other cultures, e.g., the ancient Chinese, Greeks, and Magyars, also expressed their beliefs and ideas about alcohol in their folk medical practices. Keller also traces the development of various antidotes to alcoholism, from Old Testament to contemporary days, which can be broadly categorized into abstinence or aversion techniques. The underlying assumption behind various aversion techniques is that the alcoholic does not want to give up his or her drinking.

Keller demonstrates that for centuries alcoholism treatment was carried out purely on an ad hoc basis. There was no scientific or systematic approach to alcoholism. Treatment was idiosyncratic, not systematic or rational. This perhaps is true even today, although most treatment programs use the overall blueprint of the Yale alcoholism treatment programs. Despite all the scientific debates and research over what constitutes "alcoholism" and how best to treat it, as Keller's article notes, there still exists considerable controversy.

Keller points out the difficulty in separating the medical from the behavioral treatment for alcoholism—the physical from the social consequences. Hence, the Yale Center's multifaceted approach and treatment regimen (individual psychotherapy, religious and vocational counseling, and involvement in and with AA) has become the model for most contemporary alcoholism treatment programs. Keller also suggests that the prevalent substitution of group for individual therapy in most threatment programs may have been the consequence of forces external to the needs of alcoholics—a shortage of therapeutically trained personnel and the subscription to the AA model and its assumptions regarding group support.

Keller also raises the controversial topic of spontaneous remission from drinking, a topic in which interest was sparked especially by the publication of the Rand Report (Armor et al., 1975). He notes (this volume) that some alcoholics appear to suddenly stop drinking—something that was understood as early as 1876 by Dr. T. C. Crothers. Keller points out that there still exists very little understanding of this process of spontaneous remission among alcoholics.

Mark Lender focuses on the impact of ideology (as expressed in the cultural definition of women's role in society) on our understanding and treatment of women alcoholics. Lender claims that the special stigma attached to alcoholic women is the result of the idealogy and certain socioeconomic realities of the nineteenth-century that resulted in various latent consequences for women alcoholics—hidden alcoholism, resultant ill health, delay or avoidance of treatment, and "covering up" on the part of family members. He argues that the cultural ideology regarding gender roles and stigma of women's alcoholism contributed to this special problem (see Schur, 1984).

The societal images and definitions of what women were supposed to be and the cultural assumptions of the effect of alcohol on women contributed to the denial of alcoholism among women. Thus, the ideology of the past century continues to determine views of alcoholism among women.

Women were portrayed as the guardians of family sanctity and future generations; they were the paragons of conscience (bringing up children in a Christian manner, embodying love and loyalty) and conduct (exhibit self-control, provide role models, and maintain a well-kept home), and were expected to actively express and work to ensure these domestic roles. Thus, the popular image and expectation of an ideal woman and the stereotype of an alcoholic were incompatible. Alcoholic parents are described as neglectful and abusive to their children. Moreover, the various vignettes Lender cites demonstrate the belief that alcoholic parents were not exclusively the poor, but were distributed across the social class spectrum.

During the nineteenth century, the pivot of middle-class social life was not the individual but the nuclear family that had come to replace the old institutions—the corporate village and extended family of the colonial era. And women's social status was an extension of their familial role. The nuclear family came to exemplify independence and individual responsibility, norms that were suitable to an expanding, competitive post-revolutionary economy. There was a general antipathy toward alcoholics; however, a drunken woman was considered worse than a drunken man. Norms regarding women's sexual and familial roles were more exacting than those for men; and therefore women who engaged in deviant drinking were perceived as deviating from their gender and familial roles. They were depicted as having lost their motherly interests, and various unseemly sexual activities, such as promiscuity, incest, prostitution, pimping, and being victims of white slavery, were attributed to them.

Curiously, women alcoholics were also accused of driving men to drink. Evidently, nineteenth-century Americans could not conceive of the reverse phenomenon! The wide appeal of the temperance movement was not just due to an antipathy toward alcohol per se, but also to the popular perception that alcohol posed a threat to the central values revolving around the nuclear family and with a concern for future generations. It is not surprising that since a woman's social existence hinged on her familial-role performance, a network of supportive services for alcoholic women was lacking. Those who hid their alcoholism or received treatment secretly had a better chance of retaining their social status. However, not all strata of society could afford such treatment or had the privacy. Moreover, the ideology was rampant with negativism concerning a woman alcoholic's ability to abstain from alcohol. Worse still, the professional's medical view, portraying women as the "weaker sex" and having a "nervous organization that was susceptible to alcohol," reflected this popular conception. One can only wonder what self-fulfilling prophecies these ideas created!

Gail Milgram's article deals with the founding and growth of the Summer School of Alcohol Studies—still the major training center for professionals in the fields of alcohol treatment, education and treatment training. Within two years of the end of Prohibition, the beginnings of the "alcoholism movement" emerged in embryonic form and much of the basic infrastructure of the movement was well established within the first decade or so.

According to Milgram (this volume), the future Center of Alcohol Studies (CAS) evolved from two separate sources during the middle 1930s: (1) Dr. Jolliffe, chief of medical services of the psychiatric division of Bellevue Hospital in New York City, while treating alcoholics for alcohol-related illnesses decided that more scientific knowledge was needed about alcoholism per se, rather than only medical complications resulting from it. Accordingly, he designed an interdisciplinary study of alcoholism and in 1937 organized the Scientific Advisory Commission (later called the Research Council on the Problems of Alcohol). (2) Two of the people in the Commission were researchers at the Laboratory of Applied Physiology at Yale University. One, Dr. Yandell Henderson, had been studying the nature of intoxication; another, Dr. Howard Haggard, had been studying the metabolism and effects of alcohol.

The Research Council received a grant, hired Jellinek, and Jellinek was invited by Haggard to join the Yale staff (see Keller, this volume). Thus, the Section of Studies on Alcohol was founded within the Laboratory of Applied Physiology. This soon became a separate unit, called the Center of Alcohol Studies (CAS), headed by Haggard.

The SSAS was founded in 1943. In 1944, one of its students, Mrs. Marty Mann, founded the National Committee for Education on Alcoholism (now known as the National Council on Alcoholism). In 1945, the first of the outpatient alcoholism clinics, known as

Yale Plan Clinics, encompassing research as well as a variety of treatments, was founded. Also initiated by the CAS in the mid-1940s was an industry program for treating employed alcoholics and the American Association for Instruction on Alcohol and Narcotics to stimulate changes in education about alcohol. Thus, the CAS became a center of publication, education, research, and treatment, and stimulated other organizations carrying on these activities.

The CAS and SSAS educational activities grew and changed in a milieu of growing public awareness of alcohol problems and of the need for treatment, research, education, and treatment-training. Although initially there was a single curriculum for the four weeks of SSAS, in 1948 two separate curricula were offered during the second two weeks: one for people in education and law enforcement and another for physicians, social workers, and others directly involved in treatment. In 1949 a three-week western session was offered in San Antonio but was later discontinued.

Other developments in the field of alcoholism treatment and research were the founding, in 1949, of the Alcoholism Research Foundation of Ontario (which was to become the Addiction Research Foundation) and of the National States' Conference on Alcoholism (this became the North American Association of Alcoholism Programs in 1956 and the Alcohol and Drug Problems Association in 1972). In 1951 Al-Anon (for wives and other close adults of alcoholics) and the North Conway Institute (to draw clergy into ministering to alcoholics) were started. In 1957 Alateen (for the teenage children of alcoholics) was founded.

The CAS, with its director, Selden D. Bacon, a sociologist, moved to Rutgers University in 1962. The clinical function of the Yale Center was suspended at this point. Funding was obtained both from the National Institute of Mental Health and the Smithers Foundation. In 1963 professional qualifications and college education or equivalent experience were explicitly set forth as admissions requirements for the SSAS applicants.

The format of the SSAS was changed in 1964 to become even more specialized; each student, in addition to attending general seminars, took two special (out of a possible thirteen) courses. The same year, a separate two-week "Physicians' Institute" and a one-week "Northeast Institute" for those whose activities were only tangential to alcohol problems were organized, but these continued only until 1969.

In 1975 the SSAS started offering courses on abuse of drugs other than alcohol. In collaboration with the New Jersey State Department of Health and the Prudential Insurance Company, the SSAS initiated the New Jersey Summer School of Alcohol and Drug Abuse in 1976. Thus, a state governmental agency and private enterprise became jointly involved in alcohol treatment.

The general tendencies of the SSAS from 1943 to the present have been as follows: first, an increase in the number of courses offered (from eight to forty); second, growth in the variety of disciplines encompassed in these; third, greatly increased specialization of courses; fourth, increasing proportion of college graduates among the students; fifth, a change in student body from those whose knowledge of alcoholism was tangential to their vocation to professionals whose prime focus is on alcoholism treatment.

Sheila Blume's article covers a more recent period, alcoholism treatment in the 1950s in New York State. She too demonstrates how societal factors affected attitudes toward and the treatment of alcoholics in general, and of women in particular. As Blume points out, even in a 1,000-bed hospital there were no systematic or organized treatment programs for alcoholism per se.

The level of knowledge of medical professionals during this period was generally limited to description of individual alcoholic patients and their behavior; most often, these patients were admitted into the medical facility for something other than alcoholism. The only characteristic noted in classifying and treating alcoholics was that of gender. Information on other aspects of alcoholism was not only scarce, but also reflected the negative and condescending attitudes of the professionals. Psychiatrists were involved in treating lobotomized schizophrenics, but not alcoholics.

The stigma attached to alcoholics—the "morally defunct"—was very strong. The social milieu of the 1950s was mirrored even in the attitudes of those few interested in treating alcoholics, reflecting their assumption that the alcoholic needed only the will and desire to stop consuming alcohol. And there were other barriers that blocked the development of systematic alcoholism treatment—lack of economic and political power of most alcoholics.

The stigma attached to alcoholics—the "morally defunct"—was very strong. The social milieu of the 1950s was mirrored even in the attitudes of those few interested in treating alcoholics, reflecting their assumption that the alcoholic needed only the will and desire to stop consuming alcohol. And there were other barriers that blocked the development of systematic alcoholism treatment—lack of economic and political power of most alcoholics.

The perception of alcoholism as a reflection on one's moral failure or failure of "will" changed to that of a curable disease, but only gradually. Increasingly, admitting one's alcoholism became less of a threat to one's respectability. Not only did professional groups and institutions become increasingly involved in dealing with alcoholism, but the 1950s Republican and Democratic parties in New York State included in their platforms the definition of alcoholism as a disease and a public health problem. Thus, political factors contributed to the passage of various statutes and state-level programs for alcohol problems. The idea that alcoholism is a social problem rather than an individual, idiosyncratic defect emerged, echoing once again the ideology of the temperance era.

During the 1960s, several new trends emerged in alcoholism treatment. Psychiatry residents' training in alcoholism was influenced by the prevalent ideology of their teachers—negativism and a sense of futility. The only program specifically oriented to alcoholic patients was AA, with voluntary attendance, in the male wards of psychiatric hospitals. By default, Blume (no one else wanted the job) assumed charge of an experimental male alcoholism unit (stigmatized and labeled "the country club") that was open, voluntary, and organized with the goal of encouraging morale and group spirit.

Blume decided to create an alcoholism therapy group among the women patients and based the new program on her readings of the limited literature that existed. Most of the research literature described male alcoholics.

Blume, influenced by Al-Anon, incorporated AA volunteers, used psychodrama, integrated pastoral counseling, involved the community and other groups into the treatment unit. In this manner, the audience and constituency for alcoholism treatment were expanded. By requiring psychiatric residents to spend some time among alcoholics, Blume influenced the image of alcoholism that these residents entertained. Media attention during the 1960s helped improve the image of treatment programs and personnel, and raised the morale of the practitioners. Consequently, the public perception of alcoholism and ideas regarding it also changed.

A new alcoholism treatment unit was founded in New York State in 1965. Various state agencies became involved in this program and a network of seventeen inpatient units in the State was created. In 1971, the New York State Research Unit on Alcoholism came into being. The political and social climate of the times permitted such innovation and expansion of human services. In 1978 the Alcoholism Division of New York State broke away from the Mental Health Unit, thereby establishing legitimacy, power, and credibility for alcoholism treatment as a distinctly different discipline from other mental health fields. This entity became a rallying point for diverse alcoholism constituencies.

Now that we have examined the historical development of alcoholism treatment, we shift our attention to the analysis of some specific treatment programs and issues.

Contemporary Programs

Florence Andrew's article reveals the effects of the unplanned interaction in an institution where public inebriates were confined. She observed and interviewed the staff and inmates in a county workhouse in a metropolitan area that housed about 100 inmates, most of whom were convicted of midemeanors and a third of whom were public drunkenness offenders.

One of the latent effects of being a public inebriate was that these offenders provided, without any security risks, a dependable and free source of labor for the institutions. In spite of lack of medical support and help, the staff quite competently anticipated, monitored, and managed the delirium tremens (DT) among their charges. The lack of medical support and help was due to the fact that the hospitals in the area refused to admit the DT cases and the attending staff physician could spend only an hour a day at the institution.

There was a mutuality in the interaction between the institutional staff and those sentenced to the workhouse. For example, the "regulars" used the institution as their mailing address. There were other aspects to this relationship—an informal bond developed between the "guarded" and the "guards," demonstrating that in any total institution such unanticipated relationships can emerge. The institution was a positive experience for most of the alcoholic inmates. It provided clean, warm, and safe shelter, nutritious food, moderate outdoor work, and an opportunity to learn farming and mechanical skills. When the inmates were released, the staff went out of their prescribed, bureaucratic roles by arranging for jobs and shelter and often gave some of their personal funds to those being discharged since the institution did not provide for post-release care.

These revelations raise several issues. What is the role of nonprofessional staff in such institutions? What are the consequences of availability or nonavailability of aftercare for people confined in institutions for alcohol problems? After all, it can be argued that a total institution is less threatening to sobriety than being let loose without the support network or resources, given the uncertainties of the larger society.

Miriam Rodin et al. discuss both similarities and differences between the findings of their study of Skid Row alcoholics in Illinois and earlier studies of other investigators (Wiseman, 1970) conducted prior to the Uniform Detoxification Act of 1976 which decriminalized public intoxication in many states.

The earlier studies show that Skid Row alcoholics made use of, with varying degrees of preference and coercion, primarily institutional resources such as mental hospitals, jails and missions. These and other institutions provided food, lodging, and other material needs in exchange for varying degrees of temporary restriction of the liberties of those who attend them, including attempts to "reform" them.

Important changes have taken place in Skid Row during the 1970s. First, voluntary detox centers have replaced mental hospitals and jails as temporary havens where homeless alcoholics could find the immediate necessities of life. Though the nature of the resources has changed, the authors found that those on Skid Row have, just as they had earlier in dealing with the staff of other institutions, learned to manipulate the staff of detox centers. Unfortunately, as several other investigators have found, the "revolving door" in and out of detox centers have been spinning faster than the jail doors previously. Second, since 1970 other needy clientele (the deinstitutionalized mental patients, the homeless, drug abusers, welfare mothers with children) have moved into Skid Row and compete with alcoholics for the limited public services available. Third, there is more violence on Skid Row. Older alcoholics are more vulnerable to attacks by younger drug abusers looking for means of supporting their habit.

The authors feel that their data illustrate the "game playing" that occurs between recidivist public inebriates and those who are supposed to serve them. Between 1977 and 1982, they find numerous indications that the staff of the 24 detox centers in Illinois have developed a certain resistance to admitting chronic "repeaters" (10+ admissions). The number of "repeaters" peaked in 1978 and declined 62 percent by 1982. Police cooperation also decreased;

transportation of "repeaters" to detox shelters peaked in 1979 and decreased 51 percent by 1982.

On the other hand, they feel their data indicate that persistence on the part of public inebriates pays off. The strongest predictor of readmissions to detox was the number of prior admissions! Other strong correlates were being homeless and having a high social problems score. Being unemployed and unmarried had smaller correlations with readmissions.

Interviews with twenty directors of detox centers reveal pessimism regarding the usefulness of their attempts to steer recidivists to rehabilitation programs. Almost half of those interviewed favored reintroducing involuntary components with regard to treatment. An equal number favored voluntary shelters and "wet hotels" rather than "treatment" in the medical sense, as well as a preference for a shift from the currently dominant "disease model" to a social model of creating community structures to envelope recidivists in new lifestyles over a long period of time.

Earl Rubington's article addresses a number of questions: (1) Do public detoxes try to get their clients to stay on? (2) How do detox staffs affect readmissions? (3) How do detox personnel influence client post-detox referrals?

From observations in six public detox centers, Rubington provides evidence of their efforts to control client's retention and readmission rates, to counsel clients, and of the relationships between these and post-detox referrals. He concludes that the failure of public detoxes to achieve the goals that alcoholism policy reformers had projected for them can be understood by examining social milieus in conjunction with clients' characteristics.

Since the length of stay in treatment has a direct effect on sobriety, the staff try to control this factor in various ways: (1) gatekeepng at the intake level by "administratively" rejecting the multiple repeaters, (2) forcing clients into post-detox referral when the client violates an "informal" contract to stay sober his/her way, (3) refusing admission on grounds of security to those already labeled "troublemakers," and (4) biased evaluations by staff based on personal likes and dislikes of certain clients.

He focuses on the internal processes in, and the external influence on, such treatment facilities, their adaptation to the constraints they face, given the mixed and somewhat contradictory roles they perform. External factors, such as legislation requiring admission, limit their control over the selection and retention of clients (while in private-treatment programs, such decisions are within the purview of the staff). Moreover, the goals of public-treatment programs are different—to help those who need it, sustain others, and change yet others. In addition, the bureaucratic structures of the organizations may themselves create tensions and strains.

Rubington points out that treatment outcome may also be a function of the internal dynamics of the treatment programs. He argues that the degree of routinization of the client-counselor interaction has an effect on the outcome. However, the degree of routinization is a product also of social and historic factors.

The author uses five indices of routinization: (1) the counselor-client ratio, (2) the proportion of counselors who are themselves recovering alcoholics, (3) the number of years of counseling experience the staff had, (4) the amount and depth of information the counselors collect on clients, and (5) the amount of time counselors spend with their clients. The amount of time counselors spend with their clients is dependent on the degree of professionalization and the ideological commitment of the staff, and the demands of bureaucratic chores such as filling out forms.

As publicly funded facilities, these detox units must demonstrate their effectiveness. Sometimes this accountability is expressed in terms of occupancy rates. However, environmental factors such as location determine occupancy rates. When whites were brought in for treatment as a last resort to a detox unit located in a black neighborhood the whites promptly checked themselves out within 24 hours. Being under pressure to maintain a certain level of occupancy, these treatment facilities may use a lenient readmission policy which in turn may affect the length of stay and the "cure" rate. Thus outcome may be solely determined by factors beyond the control of the treatment facility and its staff.

Rubington concludes with a typology of detox cultures and suggests changes which may simplify the detox process, raise the staff morale and possibly even improve outcomes. He points out that the detox staff use the available organizational resources—the experience of working with a variety of detox clients—in coping with the key problems of readmission, retention, counseling, and resolution of policy conflicts. Unfortunately, as many of the articles in this volume seem to suggest, bureaucratic needs seem to receive priority over clients' needs. That is, the manifest function of these treatment facilities become secondary to the latent, organizational ones.

External factors, such as the low professional esteem associated with treating alcoholics (not unique to this group of service personnel), has serious consequences. Moreover, being publicly funded projects, these treatment programs are legally required to admit anyone who seeks admission. This means that, theoretically, the staff has no control over whom they can admit, thereby becoming the "dumping ground" for hopeless cases whose prognoses are bleak. These clients' low social statuses rub off on the treatment personnel who are at the same time subject to tripartite allegiance— the institution, the profession, and the clients.

Melvin Tremper's article also examines the roles of factors external to the treatment setting and extraneous to the treatment regimen that create strains for the treatment personnel who rely on an ideology of patients' "motivation" and "dependence" to explain patients' behavior. The concept of motivation, according to Tremper, helps the staff select those whom they wish to admit, and the concept of dependence helps staff cope with demands of clients in bureaucratic situations of multiple lines of authority and conflicting role demands.

Tremper is skeptical about the staff's concepts of patients' "motivation" and "dependency". He points out that they are rationalizations by which lower-level staff personnel give short shrift to patients' needs because of excessive demands made by higher-up echelons (and two separate lines at that). He suggests that such an ideology is possible only in the absence of standardized treatment techniques, the effectiveness of which can be objectively assessed. These deficiancies permit personnel to make arbitrary decisions regarding patients and interpretations of their behaviors. One wonders if conflicting role demands and lines of authority and low prestige of treatment personnel would continue if techniques of treatment and evaluation were much more advanced than they are at present.

Tremper also suggests that the bureaucratic red tape involved in meeting simple requests by patients (e.g., making a phone call, buying some cigarettes) actually creates the very "dependency" that the staff righteously bemoan.

Joan Volpe and James Rooney's article is based on participant observation of a halfway house for women alcoholics, modeled after a program for male alcoholics, staffed by both recovering alcoholics and nonalcoholics. The male director in charge of both the men's and women's halfway houses was himself a recovering alcoholic.

The goals of the facility were to provide shelter for and counseling to recovering alcoholic women and to integrate them into the AA subculture. The women went to this facility quite voluntarily, but most of them had very low levels of social and economic resources and had no other place to go. In theory, it was an ideal setting—small in size, with simple rules and with low levels of status differentiation. In fact, it came close to what Goffman (1961) referred to as "a total institution."

For several years the facility was divided into two hostile factions. On one side were a recovering-alcoholic director, a tyrannical cook who acted as a spy for the director, and some of the residents. This faction, the "insiders," felt that non-alcoholic professionals did not have a useful role to play in alcoholism treatment (only AA and sharing of experiences by recovering alcoholics were considered appropriate treatment). On the other side were a succession of managers (usually not recovering alcoholics; there was rapid turnover; they were hired by a board of managers but could be fired by the director) and some of the residents. This faction, the "outsiders," felt that non-alcoholic professionals also had a useful role to play in alcoholism treatment.

"Insiders" were allowed to break rules; "outsiders" were maligned. Since most of the residents had no other place to go, "outsiders," against their better judgment, often behaved in a way that was contradictory to their understanding of the AA philosophy of honesty and integrity to which they subscribed. They overlooked gross infractions of rules by outsiders and were not candid in discussion and meetings. A typology of coping strategies by "outsiders" is presented by the authors, using Goffman's (1961) ideas on the social organization of total institutions.

The cook-tyrant castigated those who disagreed with her as not having the proper "motivation." When some outsiders finding the place unbearable, left prematurely, this was considered further proof of their lack of "motivation." And when some of those returned to drinking, this was yet more proof of no "motivation."

S. Priyadarsini's paper is based on participant observation in a private, coed facility for alcoholics. The residents were more or less a homogeneous group—white and middle class. The therapeutic facility was a small, mostly residential facility that required a minimum of four weeks' stay. Its program consisted of the following treatment processes—individual and (sex-segregated and coed) group therapy, education, and linkup with AA.

Whatever may be the causes and cures of alcoholism, the conduct of alcoholics is an extension of their respective gender roles in society. Research and literature in the field of alcohol studies suggest that there are gender-based differences in the characteristics, behavior, and prognoses of alcoholics. However, treatment processes and techniques tend to ignore these differences. Moreover, treatment seems to be based on the personnel's assumptions regarding male alcoholics and their needs.

The author's observations on this treatment program also suggest that there may be differences between men and women alcoholics insofar as they differed in (1) the amount of initiative each took in group sessions, (2) the topics and issues that seemed to concern each, (3) their degree of formality of demeanor and language, and (4) the level of affectivity each exhibited in therapeutic sessions. The researcher found that the male alcoholic residents lived up to the cultural ideology regarding males—they initiated the discussions in coed sessions while the women, even in single-gender sessions, had to be prodded to participate, let alone initiate discussions. Male patients' behavior was reflective, in yet another way, of their gender role. They tended to focus on the nature of their work, problematic relationships with bosses and coworkers and their effects on sobriety, as well as quitting, finding and changing jobs. The women, on the other hand, were concerned with the cultural expectations of women as nurturing and emotional. They talked about expressing their honest feelings and emotions in interpersonal relations and social networks.

The women, with regard to propriety, tended to be more formal in manner, language, and appearance whether in single-gender or coed sessions. Men "let their hair down" more often in coed as well as single-gender sessions. The men freely used "four-letter" words (which embarrassed the women) and were more openly and blatantly critical of the facility and each other. However, the women were more demonstrative and affectionate in their behavior while men were more detached and "calm." The implications of these gender-based differences for alcoholism treatment are discussed by the author.

REFERENCES

Armor, D. et al. *Evaluating Alcoholism Treatment* (Santa Monica, Calif.: The Rand Corp., 1975).

Clark, N.H. *Deliver us From Evil: An Interpretation of American Prohibition* (N.Y.: Norton and Co., 1976).

Conrad, P. and J.W. Schneider *Deviance and Medicalization: From Badness to Sickness* (St. Louis, Missouri: Mosby, 1980).

Edwards, G. et al. "Alcoholism: A Controlled Trial of 'Treatment' and 'Advice,' *Journal of Studies on Alcohol* 38(5): 1004-1031, 1977.

Goffman, E. *Asylums: Essays on the Social Situation of Mental Patients and Other Inmates* (Chicago: Aldine, 1961).

Gusfield, J. *Symbolic Crusade: Status Politics and the American Temperance Movement* (Urbana, Ill.: University of Illinois Press, 1963).

Lender, M. and J.K. Martin *Drinking in America* (London: Macmillan, 1982).

Levine, H.G. "The Discovery of Addiction: Changing Conceptions of Habitual Drunkenness in America," *Journal of Studies on Alcohol* 39(1): 143-174, 1978.

Levine, H.G. "The Alcohol Problem in America: From Temperance to Alcoholism," *British Journal of Addiction* 79: 109-119, 1984.

Schneider, J.W. "Deviant Drinking as Disease: Alcoholism as a Social Accomplishment" *Social Problems* 24: 361-372, 1978.

Schur, E.M. *Labeling Women Deviant: Gender, Stigma, and Social Control* (N.Y.: Random House, 1984).

Weiner, C.L. *The Politics of Alcoholism: Building an Arena Around A Social Problem* (New Brunswick, N.J.: Transaction Books, 1981).

Wiseman, J.P. *Stations of the Lost* (Chicago: University of Chicago, 1979).

The Old and the New in the Treatment of Alcoholism

Mark Keller

If we are to speak of the treatment of alcoholism the first question we must resolve is, what is it that we contemplate treating. What is the nature of the condition? From my viewpoint, we talk about treatment for alcoholism, first, because we regard alcoholism as a disease.

There has been some confusion on this issue in recent times. Some people who are interested in alcoholism and concerned about it have questioned whether it is properly classified as a disease. One way in which the confusion is manifested is the popularization of the term "alcohol abuse." If you hear me use that abusive term, you may be sure it is only in quotation marks. I don't use it because I don't know what it is and I am not sure when others use it that they know what it is. The confusion arises from the fact that alcoholism is obtrusively marked by gross repeated intake of alcohol to the point of intoxication. Now intoxication with alcohol is often achieved by a lot of people all over the world who are not alcoholics—that is, who do not have the disease alcoholism. They drink to drunkenness for a great variety of reasons which I will not discuss now, though it is useful to note that some of them are drinking that way because they have entered the process of becoming alcoholics. They are learning to be alcoholics. But many people cannot distinguish or don't want to distinguish between those who voluntarily or accidentally get drunk sometimes and sometimes get into trouble on account of it, and others who repeatedly get drunk because they cannot help it, and because they are addicted to the drug alcohol. By using the same kind of descriptive label—whether alcoholism or the pejorative label "alcohol abuse"—for both kinds of people, they confuse

This paper is revised from a lecture delivered at the International Congress on Alcoholism, Jerusalem, 21-26 September, 1981.

The author is Emeritus Professor of Documentation, the Center of Alcohol Studies, Rutgers University, New Brunswick, New Jersey.

themselves to the degree that they think all who get drunk are alcoholics, or all of them are mere misbehavers, and so they are able to deny that there is a disease alcoholism. Perhaps, as a World Health Organization group suggested a few years ago, we ought to abandon the now confused term alcoholism and call the condition alcohol-dependence syndrome (Edwards, et al., 1977). I, for one, would prefer to speak of alcohol addiction. I think I can justify classifying a drug addiction as a disease. But if I know anything about language, about terminology, about usage, I know that we are not going to give up "alcoholism." It seems to be a word with more magic in it than abracadabra.

Let us at least remember, then, that there are people who have a diagnosable disease, alcohol addiction or alcoholism, and other people who also sometimes get drunk but are not addicted. In discussing treatment of alcoholism I shall be talking about those who do have the disease. And I shall therefore speak of them as patients, not clients.

One more preliminary note about alcoholism as a disease is worth adumbrating: nowadays a lot of people imagine that the idea of alcoholism as a disease is something new, discovered or invented in America relatively recently, in the 1940s. This is an error due to ignorance of history. In recorded history there never was a time when alcoholism was not recognized and treated as a disease. Dr. T. D. Crothers (1882) refers to such recognition in ancient Egyptian papyri and quotes Herodotus, Diodorus and Plutarch to the same effect and I have traced it to the Bible and the Talmud (Keller, 1976). It's true that at some times and in some places some people did not understand that some of the people who were repeatedly and catastrophically getting drunk had a disease. It's true that at some times and in some places the disease concept was nearly—but not completely—forgotten. That was especially likely to happen when the dominant feeling was to solve the problems around alcohol by means of severely restrictive laws. That is what happened in America and elsewhere in the latter 19th and early 20th centuries during the victorious march of the Classical Temperance Movement toward prohibition (Bacon, 1967; Keller, 1982). But when the extreme legislative policies were seen to have failed, the reality of alcoholism as disease was newly popularized and that gave the erroneous impression of a new discovery or of a policy-inspired invention.

With these preliminaries out of the way I can begin tracking some of the historic facts about the treatment of alcoholism. The earliest recorded methods may seem primitive. The friends and relatives of the drunkard were advised to put a worm or insect into his wine. This, it was hoped, might create a disgust for the beverage. Another ancient remedy was to load everything the drunkard ate and drank with wine. This too was supposed finally to make him so disgusted with the taste that he would give it up entirely. If these attempts strike us as more folk-medicine than science, we may nevertheless recognize in them the beginnings of some very modern conditioning methods. There are no ancient medical records to tell us that any alcoholics were ever cured by these treatments. But in modern times I have observed—and friends in the medical profession confirm me in this—that almost any method ever tried in treating alcoholism has some success. For example, I know of a man, by profession an electrical engineer, who thought alcoholism could be treated by limiting the patient to monocular vision. He had quite an elaborate neuro-electrical theory to account for this hypothesis. Moreover, he cured his own alcoholism by permanently wearing a patch over one eye. So, it seems not unreasonable to assume that the classical worm-in-wine and the alcoholic-hypersaturation treatments achieved some success.

The challenge to the disease concept of alcoholism has been accompanied, sometimes from the same sources, by a challenge to the idea that the only appropriate goal of treatment for alcoholism is permanent total abstinence. Here again an error due to ignoring history helps to confuse the issue. At least some of those who challenge the abstinence goal imagine that it is an invention of Alcoholics Anonymous made in the mid-1930s. If they would read the classical alcoholism literature they would find literally scores of articles dealing with alcoholism and its treatment in the burgeoning medical literature of the 19th century, articles assuming or explicitly stating that it is a disease and a public-health problem, and assuming that the "cure" of alcoholism was permanent total abstinence.

To me it seems that the idea that the safe goal for alcoholics is total abstinence is already indicated in the Bible. I will ask you to recall the story of Hannah in the first chapter of the First Book of Samuel. Hannah was childless and extremely unhappy on account of it. At the annual family pilgrimage to the shrine in Shiloh she could not partake of the festal meal. She went off by herself and stood, leaning against the wall of the shrine, praying to God to grant her a son. She prayed silently—only her lips were moving but she made no sound. Eli, the high priest, noticed her odd behavior and mistook this gentlewoman for a hallucinating drunkard. The text clearly indicates that he took her not merely to be drunken but to be a drunkard. What he said to her, in reproval and by way of prescription, confirms this understanding. He said, "How long (or 'until when') will you be intoxicating yourself." (Ad mathai tishtakarin!) Clearly he assumed that it was her customary way, that she was "one of those"—what we today would call an alcoholic. And then he prescribed for her—and let us remember that in those times the priests were also the doctors. His prescription was: "Remove (or 'get rid of') your wine from yourself!"

For those who know the classical Hebrew I will quote the exact words of the original, which are not always well translated. Eli said, "Hasiri eth yeynekh me-alayikh!" I cannot imagine a more definite prescription for total removal of drink from the person addressed. And I infer from this that such was Eli's understanding, that an addicted alcoholic must give up drink altogether.

The goal of permanent total abstinence for alcoholics is, then, an ancient expectancy. Whether it is the only practical and safe goal for all alcohol addicts is a subject that may be discussed objectively among therapists and theorists. But they should not assume that it is a new notion introduced in the 20th century by Alcoholics Anonymous and their medical friends.

The earliest recorded treatments, as I have noted, may seem primitive. Pliny the elder, in his *Historia Naturalis* (xxxii, 49), written in the 1st century, asserts that an aversion to wine may be produced in a drunkard by putting a roach or worm or other disgusting creature into his drink. Elsewhere in the same work he records that screech-owl's eggs, given in wine to a drunkard for 3 days, will cure him of the taste for drink. Variants of the worm-in-wine treatment appear repeatedly over time. A book published in England in 1601 recommends, for weaning the uncontrolled drinker of his addiction, a tonic wine in which eels have been suffocated (Lupton, 1601). If eels were not available, green frogs caught around springs would serve as well. The Chinese used both human cerumen and the head of a rat ashed in the first moon as medicaments for the treatment of alcoholism (Read, 1976). In more recent times, as recorded by von Hovorka and Kronfeld (1908-09) in their work on folk-medicine, the Ruthenians regarded pouring the drunkard's own urine back into his mouth an efficacious remedy, while the Magyars believed drunkards could be cured by secretly mixing sparrow's dung into their brandy.

The idea of secretly doctoring the alcoholic's drink undoubtedly arose from the common observation that the last thing an alcoholic wants is to be cured—that is, if it means giving up his drink. The secret-medicine method was so popular in the 19th century that newspapers were filled with advertisements of sure-cure pills and liquids that a wife could surreptitiously add to the husband's coffee. There are places where the practice survives to this day. In a recent report from Brazil, Dr. Jandira Masur and colleagues (1981) cite newspaper advertisements of medicines, obtainable without prescription from pharmacies, to be added surreptitiously to an alcoholic's diet, and sure to render him incapable of continuing to drink alcohol. The magical ingredient in this case is either ipecac or disulfiram or a mixture of both. The advertisements do not warn that this may be a cure-or-kill treatment.

Perhaps the most curious of the surreptitious treatments of alcoholism is one reported by von Hovorka and Kronfeld (1908-09) from Ruthenia. It consists of placing a piece of pork secretly into a Jew's bed and keeping it there 9 days, then pulverizing it and feeding it secretly to the drunkard. He will then, it is believed, abhor alcoholic drink as a Jew abhors pork.*

In the latter part of the 18th century the foremost physician in the American colonies, Dr. Benjamin Rush (1814), published a remarkable essay on what we today call alcoholism. Its title is, "An Inquiry Into the Effects of Ardent Spirits Upon the Human Body and Mind, with an Account of the Means of Preventing and of the Remedies for Curing Them." I cite this work because Doctor Rush, educated by the leading medical authorities in Europe, with extensive experience in Philadelphia and as a Surgeon-General of the American Revolutionary Army, was as well informed as any physician of his time.

I may note first as a matter of historical interest that Doctor Rush wrote of chronic drunkenness as a disease. In fact he expressed the very modern idea that it "resembles certain hereditary, family and contagious diseases." For the treatment of "the recurrence of fits of drunkenness, and to destroy the desire for ardent spirits" Doctor Rush considered three types of measures to have been demonstrated efficacious: religious, metaphysical (what we today call psychological), and medical.

Of the use of religion he cites no specific examples but in a brief paragraph states that the acquisition of a practical belief in the doc-

---

*For most of the old and folk remedies I am indebted to the indefatigable British alcohologist of a former generation, Dr. J. D. Rolleston (1941).

trines of the prevailing religion had cured many hundred drunkards of the desire for ardent spirits. In contrast, Doctor Rush illustrates with many case reports how various sorts of psychological experiences had effected even instant cures. It is evident, however, that Rush was most impressed by the efficacy of "The association of the idea of ardent spirits with a painful or disagreeable impression upon some part of the body." He was of course too sophisticated for the worm-in-the-wine technique but was near to one of the most modern techniques based on Pavlovian principles. He reports, for example, the following case:

> I once tempted a Negro man, who was habitually fond of ardent spirits, to drink some rum (which I placed in his way) and in which I had put a few grains of tartar emetic.—The tartar sickened and puked him to such a degree, that he supposed himself to be poisoned. I was much gratified by observing he could not bear the sight nor smell of spirits for two years afterwards.

One-hundred and fifty years later, Doctor Walter Voegtlin (1940), who had not read Rush but had read Pavlov, was to develop the same idea into a systematic method using emetine to induce vomiting in association with alcohol. This treatment helped several thousand alcoholic patients to become total abstainers. Doctor Rush himself, never having heard of Pavlov, credited the idea to no less an authority than Moses when, he writes, Moses

> compelled the children of Israel to drink the solution of the golden calf (which they had idolized) in water. This solution [Rush continues], if made as it most probably was, by means of what is called hepar sulphuris, was extremely bitter, and nauseous, and could never be recollected afterwards, without bringing into equal detestation, the sin which subjected them to the necessity of drinking it.

Doctor Rush didn't know it, but he was a behavioral psychologist.

I have already noted that almost any method seems to be able to help some alcoholics. Doctor Rush mentions a few curious ones. A Philadelphia physician was cured by a strictly vegetarian diet. A lady of some means, whose expenditure for brandy alone came to a hundred pounds a year, 18th century Pennsylvania Currency, was helped by blisters to the ankles. A "notorious drunkard" was cured by a bout of the yellow fever, from which he recovered, under Doctor Rush's attendence, "with the loss of his relish for spirits."

Finally it is noteworthy that in the 1940s there was much discussion in the medical literature of the question whether alcoholics should be weaned gradually of drink or withdrawn suddenly. Doctor Rush had something to say on that subject a hundred and fifty years earlier. He wrote emphatically:

> It has been said that the disuse of spirits should be gradual; but my observations authorise me to say that persons who have been addicted to them should abstain from them *suddenly* and *entirely.* "Taste not, handle not, touch not" should be inscribed upon every vessel that contains spirits in the house of a man who wishes to be cured of habits of intemperance.

The examination of history leaves no doubt that alcoholism has always plagued humankind and that there has been no slack in the attempts to treat it. The 19th century saw the beginning of a more scientific practice of medicine, as well as the development of what was to become the specialty of psychiatry. This may explain the beginning of intensive medical interest in alcoholism and its treatment at that time. Special medical societies concerned with alcoholism were formed, the first specialized medical journals devoted to alcoholism were founded, and a number of learned books by great physicians, dealing exclusively with alcoholism and its treatment, were published—Doctor Rush's essay, from which I have quoted, being an early example. Moreover, quite a few specialized hospitals for alcoholics were founded. The therapeutic methods were as varied as the fertile minds of the therapists could devise. We might tend to think of them as mainly psychological, and indeed the practice of treating alcoholism tended increasingly to fall into the province of the developing specialty of psychiatry. There was a tendency to confine alcoholics to specialized alcoholism hospitals, called then inebriate asylums, for considerable lengths of time, as much as a year, and sometimes to general mental hospitals or sanitariums. Like all treatments, apparently the long institutional confinement also produced its fair share of remissions. Some alcoholics emerged as confirmed abstainers.

Psychological methods were not the only ones, however. Thus the famous Doctor Keeley developed his physiological treatment, not made public but presumed to consist of injections of colloidal gold, which became the basis of a flourishing business and many imitations. To my mind the most interesting and significant development in the treatment of alcoholics occurred in the early years of the present century—that is, the beginning of group therapy.

But hard times were now rapidly overtaking the therapeusis of alcoholism. The very growth of treatment for alcoholics, with institutions and professional societies and journals, was ammunition in the armory of the organized antialcohol movement (Bacon, 1967). The antialcohol movement succeeded, during the first quarter of the present century, in getting legislation adopted in many places and in whole countries which severely limited the legal availability of alcohol or even totally prohibited its manufacture or sale. The outstanding example of this process is national prohibition of alcohol by amendment of the Constitution in the United States. More or less severe prohibitions or restrictions were adopted in many other countries.

These legislative actions had a notable effect on alcoholism and on the treatment of alcoholism—notable, and curious, and ironic. At first there was a reduction in the public manifestations of alcoholism: fewer arrests for drunkenness, fewer alcoholic admissions to hospitals. The specialized alcoholism hospitals closed up, went out of business. Doctors stopped seeing alcoholic diseases. The legislative solution seemed to work and treatment of alcoholism could become an obsolete art.

The trouble was that it didn't work for very long. Some improvident alcoholics and others who did not lay up stores were deprived of alcohol for a time. But soon they found illicit sources of supply and soon the arrests for drunkenness and the hospital admissions and the alcohol-related diseases began to rise again. In a few years, the American statistics show, these indexes were at the pre-prohibition level. The movement to treat the alcoholics for their alcoholism had to wait, however, until the prohibition laws were repealed and the professions were able or forced once more to face the realities of alcoholism. It was then that medicine, including psychiatry and psychology, could rediscover alcoholism. It was then that laymen too, even alcoholics themselves, could rouse themselves to therapeutic action. So it was then that Alcoholics Anonymous was founded (Alcoholics Anonymous, 1939). It was then too that systematic research was initiated, notable in the formation of a national Research Council on Problems of Alcohol. This was followed by the development of a Center of Alcohol Studies at Yale University, the founding of a Journal of Studies on Alcohol and the first public clinics in America for the treatment of alcoholism—the Yale Plan Clinics (Keller, 1979).

Beginning in the mid-1930s, we may think of the contemporary treatment of alcoholism as generally paralleling the main streams of etiological thought on the disorder: physiological, psychological or social, and often in some combination of these viewpoints.

Let us glance first at the great variety of physiological methods. Sometimes such treatments are given as adjuncts to psychotherapy. But sometimes, especially by those who hold to strictly physiological–constitutional theories of etiology, they are given in "pure" form—that is, without conscious attempt at psychotherapy or even with an effort to avoid it. Nevertheless some proponents of purely metabolic, endocrinal, nutritional or chemical therapies recognize that psychotherapy is an unavoidable concomitant of medication.

Probably the most common drug treatment of alcoholism in recent times has been the administration of disulfiram (tetraethylthiuram disulphide). This compound has many trade names, such as Abstinyl, Antiethyl, etc., but the most common is Antabuse. The classical technique is to give the patient a daily dose of disulfiram, generally 0.5 gram, for a few days, then a small test drink of an alcoholic beverage. With disulfiram present in the body, the result of drinking alcohol is a reaction of flushing, nausea, vomiting, sudden sharp drop in blood pressure, pounding of the heart, and a feeling of impending death. These symptoms are believed to be due to an excess accumulation of acetaldehyde in the blood because disulfiram interferes with the metabolism of alcohol at the acetaldehyde stage. Without safe medical management the reaction may progress to circulatory collapse and even death. By means of the test the patient is made to experience dramatically the danger of attempting to drink while under disulfiram medication. A smaller daily dose of disulfiram in tablet form is then prescribed and the dread of the consequences of drinking is relied on to deter the alcoholic from drinking as long as he continues to take the drug. Most therapists use the period of enforced abstinence to apply psychological and rehabilitative measures that will enable the patient ultimately to abstain without the help of the chemical crutch.

In the years since Erik Jacobsen (1948) of Denmark first announced this application of the effect of disulfiram, the drug has been tried in nearly every part of the world and has gained favor with clinicians as a valuable adjunct in the treatment of alcoholic patients. Many variations of technique have been tried. Some therapists found group reaction tests advantageous; others did not subject their patients to an actual alcohol challenge but relied on verbal warnings or motion pictures of a real test to deter drinking. A number of other alcohol-reaction causing substances such as citrated calcium cyanamide, or metronidazole, have been tried occasionally as substitutes for disulfiram. The recent extraction of coprin, and its identification as 1-aminocyclopropanol, from the inkycap mushroom (*Coprinus atramentarius*) may add a new deterrent compound to this technique (Carlsson, et al., 1978).

Among physiological therapies, the conditioned-reflex treatment as developed by Dr. Walter Voegtlin (1940) on the basis of Pavlovian theory, and only slightly modified in the techniques of other therapists, has perhaps been given to more alcoholics than any other, excepting only deterrence therapy with disulfiram. This treatment is carried out in a special setting by injecting a drug, usually emetine, to induce nausea and vomiting. Precisely timed when the drug is about to take effect, the patient is given an alcoholic beverage to drink. In repeated sessions the nausea and emesis become associated with various alcoholic beverages and the patient is thus conditioned to react with aversion to the taste, smell, and even sight of them. The aversion does not last indefinitely but may be reinforced after a few months. The interval of abstinence, however, is generally used to institute psychological therapeutic and social rehabilitative measures. Apomorphine, with a different technique, has been used as the emetic by therapists in several European countries.

Other therapists have used mild electroshock as the aversive inhibitor of the alcohol-seeking. One such technique requires the patient to carry the therapeutic device on his person and shock himself whenever he thinks of taking a drink.

I am trying to describe physiological treatments. You can see how difficult—indeed, how impossible—it is to keep them separate from the psychological and the social. The very modern Pavlovian technique elaborated by Dr. Voegtlin was already understood in principle by Dr. Rush in the 18th century, and he not only found it suggested in the Bible in the Book of Exodus, but foresightedly included it among the metaphysical treatments. He, thus, regarded it as essentially psychological. What then, should we think of the most modern behavioral techniques? Obviously, being drugless, and applied mostly by psychologists, they belong in the psychological category (Marlatt and Nathan, 1978). But let us not forget their remarkable resemblance in principle to the techniques of Voegtlin, and Rush, and—putatively—Moses.

At least nutrition and hormone therapies seem to belong definitely to physiology. You may recall Dr. Rush's report of the alcoholic who was cured by a vegetarian diet. The administration of vitamins to alcoholics began only in the 1930s when it became apparent that in their "alcoholic" diseases these patients exhibited the same symptoms as those of endemic pellagra, beriberi and scurvy (Jolliffe, 1942). At that time the successful cures of deficiencies in thiamin, niacin, riboflavin, ascorbic acid and other essentials of nutrition were not mistaken for cures of the alcoholism itself. But in the 1950s, Dr. Roger J. Williams (Williams, et al., 1950) in line with his theory of the genetorophic origin of most diseases of undetermined etiology, proposed the treatment of alcoholism with massive doses of multiple vitamins. A pure test of the effectiveness of such therapy has not yet been carried out, but reports of successful nutritional treatment of some alcoholics are published occasionally.

The theory that alcoholism is caused by a disorder of endocrine function was enunciated in the 1940s and 1950s by several physicians and led to the treatment of many alcoholics with adrenal steroids and adrenocorticotropic hormone. Here again the treatments are almost invariably complicated by obvious psychotherapeutic procedures and by such factors as simultaneous affiliation with Alcoholics Anonymous. Thus the claims of specific effectiveness against alcoholism, whether of nutrition therapy or endocrinotherapy, rest on the faith of the therapist in the validity of the underlying etiological theory.

Many other physiological therapeutic measures are tried occasionally in alcoholics. Sometimes one cannot be sure from the published reports, especially when the authors write of "alcohol abuse," whether they are treating the alcoholism itself, or the chronic effects of prolonged excessive drinking, or the acute physical or so-called mental sequels of an extended spree. Among such treatments one may list intravenous injections of alcohol; injections of autoserum and alcoholized serum; antihistaminic agents; apomorphine without conditioning; carbon dioxide inhalation, neurosurgery; oxygen by injection; relaxation; strychnine; and, of course, many muscle-relaxing, tranquilizing and antidepressant drugs. In recent years acupuncture and chiropracture have been applied for alcoholism by the practitioners of those increasingly popular techniques, as well as jogging, basketball, and the oldest athletic performance—work.

In moving on to psychological therapies we should remember that the majority of psychiatrically oriented therapists see alcoholism as essentially a manifestation of personality disorder or emotional maladjustment, with roots probably in early childhood trauma. Their therapeutic methods encompass the full range of procedures employed in the treatment of the psychoneuroses and character disorders, including individual and group techniques. The aim varies from elimination of the hypothetical underlying cause to effecting just sufficient shift in the patient's emotional state so that he can function at least temporarily without recourse to drinking.

Individual treatment of alcoholics rarely takes the form of orthodox psychoanalysis, which has scored few recorded successes in alcoholism. This may be related to the comparative ease with which an alcoholic can escape the threats represented by the therapeutic process simply by getting drunk. Better success has been reported by therapists, often analytically oriented, who employ chiefly supportive techniques with the unfolding of insight gauged to the patient's individual capacity. Nevertheless the rate of success with alcoholic patients by individual psychiatry has apparently not been high and this has sometimes been attributed to the strong negative response of alcoholics to authoritative (father) figures. Only one individual technique seems to have been developed in recent times especially for the treatment of alcoholics; this involves the description by the therapist, in a first interview, of the Jellinekian phases of alcoholism (Jellinek, 1946). The aim is to gain the patient's recognition of his illness and willing acceptance of treatment, always a major hurdle with this type of patient. According to Clifton (1956) who reported good success with it, the method was first applied by Jellinek himself. It was independently discovered and found useful by Joan Jackson (1957).

Psychiatry is often combined with one of the physiological treatments and sometimes with such physical procedures as electrotherapy. It is very commonly supplemented by medication with stimulants or muscle relaxants or tranquilizers or antidepressants. It was in the early 1940s that the Yale University group with which I was then associated founded the first public outpatient clinics to specialize in the treatment of alcoholism (Jellinek, 1944). This was before we had yet adopted the name Center of Alcohol Studies and long before we moved to Rutgers University. Our idea was to use a variety of methods. We tried to fit treatments to types of patients. We treated with the classical Pavlovian conditioned-reflex method. We treated with disulfiram as soon as it became known. We treated with individual psychotherapy. We did not neglect religiotherapy and we did not overlook sociotherapy including vocational counseling, and we eagerly collaborated with Alcoholics Anonymous. But an important feature of our program was group therapy and this was first conducted by Raymond McCarthy (McCarthy, 1946). In those times we thought of Ray as a "lay therapist." Today we would probably call him an alcoholism counselor.

Our original clinics became models for outpatient alcoholism clinics throughout the U.S.A. and beyond.

The shortage of therapeutic personnel and the model of Alcoholics Anonymous may have been responsible for the widespread application of group techniques in alcoholism clinics. But it had become obvious that the therapeutic group is particularly appropriate in the treatment of alcoholism. Psychiatrists, psychologists, physicians with an interest in medical psychology, psychiatric social workers, and the many kinds of lay therapists or counselors have tried out just about every variety of group techniques. A number of interesting formal researches on problems of methodology particularly applicable to alcoholic groups were reported. I will mention a few of the early ones to illustrate the range of endeavors and progress.

Ray McCarthy (1950) published the verbatim record of a series of a series of sessions in which didactic lectures were followed by relatively superficial discussions in the group. In total contrast are the deep analytic explorations in group described by Pfeffer, Friedland and Wortis (1949). Armstrong and Gibbins (1956), in Canada, experimented with groups of various size and make-up and with methods ranging from one which the therapist assumed the role of instructor to one in which his role is that of participating member. By systematic analysis of planned variations of technique they found that therapeutic benefit could be gained in large groups of mixed gender. In their successful technique these therapists did not assume an authoritarian role, yet represented a part of the ego ideal of the patients, and symbolized certain elements in the goals of the group's core membership.

In a controlled group therapy experiment, Ends and Page (1957) treated equal groups of alcoholics either by a learning-theory, patient-centered, psychoanalytic or social-discussion technique; they thought their patient-centered method the most effective.

In another group experiment, Gliedman and his colleagues (1956) treated a number of alcoholics while the wives of the patients met in a separate group with a psychiatric social worker. The need to extend therapeutic services to the spouses or other significant relatives of alcoholics was recognized long before the current emphasis on family therapy.

Finally, Lerner (1953) and others have attempted to fill the therapeutic vacuum in the population of jailed alcoholics by means of teaching-counseling group sessions. But the usual setting of group therapy is the outpatient clinic, where it is often combined with sociotherapy or physiological treatments or both, and sometimes is supplemented by individual psychotherapy.

I am not sure I should include Alcoholics Anonymous among the group therapies. My first contact with Bill Wilson, the founding father of A.A., was in 1936, just a year after A.A. was started, and I have been in close contact with it and with many A.A.s ever since. But I still don't know just what A.A. is. I am sure it is more than group therapy. I know that most of the professionals who have treated alcoholics—and not just counselors who happen to be members of A.A.—want their patients in A.A., as that seems to be the best adjunct to any form of therapy. All I am sure of is that Alcoholics Anonymous is the best therapeutic development thus far in the realm of alcoholism, that it is the best adjunct to most professional therapies, and that for many, though not all, alcoholics A.A. alone has been a sufficient treatment. We know now that it does not work for some alcoholics who can be helped by one or other of the more formal treatments. But apparently no alcoholic is harmed by trying Alcoholics Anonymous.

In Alcoholics Anonymous one of the important factors is the spiritual element, the surrender to and reliance on a Higher Power. The spiritual element in the form of religious counseling and formal religious integration or reintegration has also been effective in the treatment of alcoholism. You may recall that this was already reported by Dr. Benjamin Rush in the 18th century (1814).

The newest in alcoholism treatment I need only to mention for the record, since they are familiar to you and are being amply described in the present sessions by their best practitioners: they are the job-related programs, confrontation techniques, the mixed-multi-approach method in which a patient is exposed to a variety of treatments simultaneously in the hope that one of them will "take," the various behavioral techniques, family therapy, and, finally, a most important modern contribution, the social-service perspective. The latter is not so much a specific therapeutic method as a wholistic way of dealing with alcoholism as a disease that impinges on a whole life and on a family and on a community, requiring coordinated, many-faceted treatment that may include social rehabilitation, a reconstitution of the way of life. This latter perspective, indeed, may explain why social work as well as Alcoholics Anonymous plays so vital a role in the successful treatment of alcoholism.

Having said so much about the history of the treatment of alcoholism I would be remiss not to say a few words about its nontreatment. Nontreatment also has results. Those results are seen in many cemeteries. But they are seen, too, in many unexplained recoveries. Already more than a hundred years ago—in 1876—Dr. T. D. Crothers, in his day probably the foremost American medical authority on alcoholism, observed that "inebriety is a self-limited disease" (1876). Some alcoholics just suddenly stop drinking, apparently without any therapeutic event. The understanding of this fortunate outcome awaits explanation. I suspect that it will be explained when we have learned a lot more than we now understand about the essential ingredients of what we call psychotherapy.

Some people are interested in history only to learn the historical names and dates. I have always thought that history has more to teach us than the bare facts that made up the past. So what is the moral of it all?

We have seen that an almost unaccountable variety of treatments of alcoholism were developed, and that many of them have about an equal rate of success. Should we learn from this—as one famous recent report (Armor, et al., 1976) suggested—that we all ought to adopt just one treatment, and that is, the cheapest? That suggestion, of course, came out of clinical inexperience, from people who were unaware how alcoholics shop around, try a variety of treatments until, individually, they find one that works for them; and how therapists, consciously and unconsciously, select patients and fit available treatments for them, and avoid patients they think they cannot help; and how the nonfit failures of one treatment setting become the fit-and-successful patients of another setting. This process probably accounts for the approximately equal so-called success rate of the different treatments. We should recognize, therefore, that the variety of treatments and therapeutic settings is beneficial in a disease with the characteristics of alcoholism.

It seems to me unavoidable to derive yet another important lesson from this history. Obviously, it would be inhumane to wait for the self-limiting factor to take care of most alcoholics. Too many perish from the disease and from its sequels and side-effects before the limit is reached. But I do not think we need to wait for the disease to start, either. You may recall that in the beginning I was careful to define alcoholism the disease as a state of confirmed alcohol addiction. But I also noted that many of those who get drunk and get into trouble thereby, who are not alcoholics, are in the process of acquiring the disease. It is reasonable to say of many of them that they are practicing and learning to become alcoholics. To me it seems that we need to learn how to intervene in that process and prevent its completion.

What I am saying is that there is reason to treat those who are in danger of acquiring the disease, those who show what Jellinek (1946) called the prodromal signs, as well as those who already have the disease. To some extent I think this is already being done. Many of the occupational programs seem to be picking up some patients who are not really addicted yet and, in effect, forcing them into treatment that will prevent completion of the process. Some of the younger people who, arrested for drunken driving, are sentenced to attend a clinical program for a term, are likely to be in the prodromal rather than in the addictive state. These programs, even if they do not yet realize it, are doing secondary prevention. But I think that more clinical programs can and should be redesigned to work with the endangered as well as with the sick. Although I have been strict in defining as disease only the condition of confirmed addiction, I do not think we need to be strict in confining the operating field of the therapeutic professions. I would hope that they would be sophisticated enough to differentiate between the endangered and the addicted, develop appropriate different treatments, and perhaps project different goals.

So go, you therapists, whether you be physicians or social workers, nurses or psychologists, counselors or psychoanalysts or clergymen, and treat the endangered as well as the addicted, treat the protoalcoholics as well as the alcoholics.

REFERENCES

Alcoholics Anonymous: The Story of How More Than One Hundred Men Have Recovered from Alcoholism (New York: Works Publishing Co., 1939).

Armor, D. J., J. M. Polich and H. B. Stanbul *Alcoholism and Treatment* (Santa Monica, Ca.: Rand Corporation, 1976).

Armstrong, J. D. and R. J. Gibbins "A Psychotherapeutic Technique with Large Groups in the Treatment of Alcoholics: A Preliminary Report," *Quarterly Journal of Studies on Alcohol* 17 (1956): 461-478.

Bacon, S. D. "The Classic Temperance Movement of the U.S.A.: Impact Today on Attitudes, Action and Research," *British Journal of Addiction* 62 (1967): 5-18.

Carlsson, A., M. Henning, P. Lindberg, P. Martinson, G. Trolin, B. Waldeck and B. Wickberg "On the Disulfirma-Like Effect of Coprine: The Pharmacologically Active Principle of *Coprinus atramentarius,"* *Acta Pharm. Tox.* 42 (1978): 292-297.

Clifton, C. S. "A Technique for the Initial Interview with Male Alcoholics," *Quarterly Journal of Studies on Alcohol* 17 (1956): 89-95.

Crothers, T. D. "Clinical Studies of Inebriety," *Medical and Surgical Reporter* 35 (1876): 125-128.

————. "History of Inebriety as a Disease," *Detroit Lancet* 5 (1882): 331-334.

Ends, E. J. and G. W. Page "A Study of Three Types of Group Psychotherapy with Hospitalized Male Inebriates," *Quarterly Journal of Studies on Alcohol* 18 (1957): 263-277.

Edwards, G., M. M. Gross, M. Keller, J. Moser, and R. Room (eds.) *Alcohol-Related Disabilities* (Geneva: World Health Organization, 1977).

Gliedman, L. H., D. Rosenthal, J. D. Frank, and H. T. Nash "Group Therapy of Alcoholics with Concurrent Group Meetings of their Wives," *Quarterly Journal of Studies on Alcohol* 17 (1956): 655-670.

Jacobsen, E. "En Medicinsk Terapi Mod Alkoholisme," ("A Medical Treatment of Alcoholism") *Nord. Med.* 40 (1948): 2062.

Jackson, J. K. "The Definition and Measurement of Alcoholism: H-Technique Scales of Preoccupation with Alcohol and Psychological Involvement," *Quarterly Journal of Studies on Alcohol* 18 (1957): 240-262.

Jellinek, E. M. "Notes on the First Half Year's Experience at the Yale Plan Clinics," *Quarterly Journal of Studies on Alcohol* 5 (1944): 279-302.

————. "Phases in the Drinking History of Alcoholics: Analysis of a Survey Conducted by the Official Organ of Alcoholics Anonymous," *Quarterly Journal of Studies on Alcohol* 7 (1946): 1-88.

Jolliffe, N. "Vitamin Deficiencies in Chronic Alcoholism," ch. III in E. M. Jellinek (ed.) *Alcohol Addiction and Chronic Alcoholism* (New Haven: Yale University Press, 1942).

Keller, M. "The Disease Concept of Alcoholism Revisited," *Journal of Studies on Alcohol* 37 (1976): 1694-1717.

————. "Mark Keller's History of the Alcohol Problems Field," *Drinking and Drug Practices Surveyor* 14 (1979): 1, 22-28.

————. "Perspective on Medicine and Alcoholism," *Alcoholism: Clinical and Experimental Research* 6 (1982): 327-332.

Lerner, A. "An Exploratory Approach in Group Counseling with Male Alcoholic Inmates in a City Jail," *Quarterly Journal of Studies on Alcohol* 14 (1953): 427-467.

Lupton, T. *A Thousand Notable Things of Sundry Sorts* (London, 1601).

Marlatt, G. A. and P. E. Nathan (eds.) *Behavioral Approaches to Alcoholism* (New Brunswick, N.J.: Rutgers University Center of Alcohol Studies, 1978).

Masur, J., J. A. Del-Porto, A. J. M. Shirakawa and D. Gattaz "Nonmedical Treatment of Alcoholism with Emetic Drugs and Disulfiram in Brazil," *Journal of Studies on Alcohol* 42 (1981): 814-818.

McCarthy, R. G. "Group Therapy in an Outpatient Clinic for the Treatment of Alcoholism," *Quarterly Journal of Studies on Alcohol* 7 (1946): 98-109.

————. "Group Therapy in Alcoholism: Transcriptions of a Series of Sessions Recorded in an Outpatient Clinic," *Quarterly Journal of Studies on Alcohol* 10 (1950): 63-108, 217-250, 479-500.

Pfeffer, A. Z., P. Friedland and S. B. Wortis "Group Psychotherapy with Alcoholics: Preliminary Report," *Quarterly Journal of Studies on Alcohol* 10 (1949): 198-216.

Read, B. E. *Chinese Materia Medica: Animal Drugs* (Taipei: Southern Materials Center, 1976).

Rolleston, J. D. "The Folk-Lore of Alcoholism," *British Journal of Inebriety* 39 (1941): 30-36.

Rush, B. *An Inquiry into the Effects of Ardent Spirits Upon the Human Body and Mind, With* an *Account of the Means of Preventing and of the Remedies for Curing Them* (Brookfield, Mass.: Merriam & Co., 1814).

Voegtlin, W. L. "Treatment of Alcoholism by Establishing a Conditioned Reflex," *American Journal of Medical Science,* 199 (1940): 802-810.

von-Hovorka, O. and A. Kronfeld *Vergleichende Volksmedizin* (Stuttgart: Strecker & Schroder; 1908-09).

Williams, R. J., L. J. Berry, and E. Beerstecher, Jr. "Genetotrophic Diseases: Alcoholism," *Texas Reports on Biology and Medicine,* 8 (1950): 238-256.

A Special Stigma:
Women and Alcoholism
in the Late 19th
and Early 20th Centuries

Mark Edward Lender

Americans traditionally have maintained different standards of acceptable social and individual behavior for men and women. Disparate gender roles have governed a host of cultural norms ranging from sexual activities to career choices, generally allowing more permissive behavior patterns among men while restricting the limits of approved conduct among women. Indeed, this phenomenon has often provided men the latitude to participate in activities that would bring strong sanctions against women. Of all the examples of this double standard, few have been more obvious than the different norms of drinking behavior for men and women. The contrast has been anything but subtle: while Americans often have dismissed occasional drunkenness in men as simply "part of growing up," or even as a symbol of masculinity, society has considered similar behavior in women as deviant. In fact, alcohol problems among women generally have carried a severe social stigma (Lisansky, 1958: 76-77; Mulford, 1977: 38). Drinking-related difficulties, as Lisansky (1958: 73) has noted, have represented "the breaking of stronger taboos against drinking and intoxication," running as they do "so strongly counter to the American ideal of self-controlled, 'ladylike' behavior."

This social stigma has been, in great measure, at the root of the so-called "hidden alcoholism" phenomenon and its medical consequences. For rather than admit to a problem which society has defined as unacceptable, women have frequently tried to hide their malady. Many have gone to extraordinary lengths in this regard, usually drinking at home or alone, and often enlisting families and friends in efforts to keep alcohol problems a secret. The social strictures against women alcoholics can be so strong, some studies have indicated, that even in Skid Row circumstances they prefer to drink alone, shunning the public drinking of men (Garrett and Bahr, 1973: 1237-1239). But the cost of this deception and sensitivity, of course, is high: health worsens as drinking continues untreated, and women often refuse help until faced with a drinking-related crisis. By this time, their physical and psychological condition is frequently worse than a male alcoholic's who apparently seeks help earlier because the stigma attached to his drinking is less. "What appears to be greater pathology in women" than in men, one review of the subject has speculated, "could be the result" not only of their drinking, but also of "the greater social disapproval and rejection associated with it" (Beckman, 1975: 800-801). If this view is correct, then social "double standards" have done more than reflect disparate public attitudes toward permissible conduct in the sexes; they have also impeded the alleviation of drinking problems in women.

While the medical and sociological facets of this special stigma against women alcoholics are now familiar, the historical aspects have received relatively scant attention. This is true even of the most basic questions, such as when the stigma first appeared, or why it evolved as it did in the United States. These are significant issues in social history (and for that matter, in medical history as well), for they reflect aspects of other important problems. Attitudes toward the social roles of women generally, early thinking on alcoholism, and the medical implications of popular beliefs, for example, are all related questions, and should remain in view in any discussion of the social sanctions against women alcoholics. Indeed, this essay will consider how these social factors initially combined to shape the special stigma, then joined with it to make "hidden alcoholism" a noteworthy issue in American medicine for the first time.

If the questions are significant, however, at least some important sources are in hand to address them. The particular problems of drinking among women attracted serious attention from the medical community and social critics by the mid-nineteenth century, and by the early twentieth century the matter had generated considerable discussion. Indeed, a sizable literature evolved, a great deal of which is now available for historical analysis. In addition to the comments of social reformers (some, but not all of whom were temperance workers), contemporary medical reports preserved a range of useful information on the physical, psychological and social aspects of alcohol problems among American women. Most of these reports were the work of physicians with particular interests in alcoholism treatment, and who generally compiled their data from patients in institutions devoted to addictions treatment in the late nineteenth and early twentieth centuries. These records, rich as they are in many cases, are insufficiently detailed for precise statistical analysis; nevertheless they are quite revealing as historical sources (Lender, 1981). This essay draws heavily on these early reports, and uses many of them in an historical context for the first time.

GENDER ROLES IN POSTBELLUM AMERICA: AN OVERVIEW

It has never been easy to generalize on American views on either sex or drinking, much less to point precisely to when specific ideas on these subjects have emerged in the popular mind. In fact, a number of careful studies have shown that feelings on both issues often have been ill-defined, with their roots tangled in a welter of concerns and ambivalence, and that in any case, they have taken shape slowly rather than gaining any sudden social preeminence. Despite these difficulties, though, we can place the origins of the stigma against women alcoholics, in substantially the form it exists today, in the last half of the nineteenth century. Moreover, its immediate roots appear to have been relatively clear: the stigma grew directly from the relationships between contemporary attitudes toward gender roles on one hand, and from public perceptions of alcoholics on the other. Thus, an understanding of both of these views is critical at the outset if we are to explain the "when" and "whys" of this special stigma.

By the mid-nineteenth century, most men and women saw gender roles more in family than in individual terms. This is a crucial point, for in the latter half of the century, at least in the eyes of the country's dominant middle classes, the nuclear family had become the repository of American values and standards of right and wrong. In this view, the preservation of the family was essential to the well-being of the republic; and thus, logically, aspects of national life that affected the family—and in particular the roles of family members (that is, gender roles)—became matters of vital public concern (Clark, 1976; Janeway, 1971; Houghton, 1957; Epstein, 1981; Bordin, 1981).

But while historians have generally agreed on the family's central position in American social thought during this period, they have been less certain as to why. The best current hypothesis holds that the family unit came to embody all the virtues inherent in the American belief in independence and individual responsibility. By the late eighteenth century, and certainly by the early nineteenth, the old institutions and symbols of communal responsibility and achievement—the corporate village of early New England, established churches, extended family structures, community-enforced behavioral norms—had all in large measure passed from the American scene. Thousands flocked West after the Revolution, or set avidly to work in the competitive atmosphere of the post-Revolutionary economy, leaving the old ways behind them forever. Taking their places was a new society of yeomen farmers and independent mechanics—self-reliant and free thinking, the classic rugged individualists and freemen of the creeds of Jefferson and Jackson. This situation, of course, was not universal in fact, nor even fully accepted intellectually; but there was also no denying the appeal of this individualistic ideal to a great deal of middle-class Americans, thousands of whom lived under precisely such circumstances (Clark, 1976; Lender and Martin, 1982).

In this society of individualists, the family was the basic social unit, and it became something sacred, to be protected against all harm. It was the family, not the community or church anymore, or even other relatives, that now shared the dangers and joys of life, that nursed sick children, that educated the young, that imparted the standards of personal conduct and of social behavior. This social order itself became traditional before the Civil War and, if anything, increased in symbolic value thereafter. For in the post-Civil War years, a host of apparent threats arose to challenge established views of the world: massive new corporations, the social dislocations born of the industrialization process—including the spread of drinking problems and the proliferation of urban saloons—and waves of new immigrants with alien religious customs, seemed poised to overwhelm American individualism. In this situation, it appeared to many citizens that a strong defense of the family, now the bastion of national values, would be the best guarantee that America could retain its old moral and social norms in the postbellum industrial world (Lender and Martin, 1982:92-93).

A number of historians have also agreed, however, that the integrity of the family depended upon its members adhering to strictly defined gender roles. And although research has detailed some remarkable variations in contemporary thought on the subject, it has also supported a contention that, by the late nineteenth century, the requirements of the middle-class family had produced a rough national consensus on what constituted an "ideal woman." It was essentially a "victorian" outlook: placed on the proverbial pedestal, women were supposed to receive the honor and protection of the rest of society; men were to shield them from the tribulations of life. This shelter, however, came at a cost. In general, women were not to compete with men in the workplace or challenge a husband's position as head of the household. Men would remain dominant in these areas while women were to function unselfishly as wives, mothers, and homemakers. A woman's joys and activities were to center on her family, and her identity and status were in the lockstep with those of her husband. In addition, her position carried a strict code of public and private morality that governed her sexual and social behavior. Society not only held women accountable to these standards, but expected her to defend and advance them; she was to be an unblemished example of morality and purity herself, and was to raise her children with the same values, thereby helping to assure their permanence. Ideally, women would live in a secure, but rigidly limited and male dominated world (Clark, 1976; Janeway, 1971; Houghton, 1957).

There were exceptions to this general view, of course: during this postwar period women were also deeply involved in a number of movements, notably women's rights and temperance. And the outlook of the Temperance Movement, for example, on the social role of women was considerably less restrictive than the general view. Too many antiliquor women had become quite active in expanding the range of opportunities open to their sex to believe that they ought to concede the leadership of society entirely to men. And in fact, many contemporaries felt that organized temperance had done more to enlarge the roles of women in all aspects of American life than any other movement in the country's history (Lender and Martin, 1982; Stewart, 1989: 9-10).

Nevertheless, even the experience of the Temperance Movement served to reinforce popular views on the role of women. Most antiliquor crusaders fully agreed that the woman's position in the home—if she voluntarily chose to stay there—was indeed special. And in this regard they even expanded on the idea that women ought to be bastions of self-control and morality. Temperance reformers saw women as the guardians of the integrity of the American family, of moral standards and of "purity." In this role they were to ensure that their children received a wholesome and Christian upbringing, to provide their husbands with love, loyalty and well-kept homes, and above all, to be the family's conscience. Moreover, this was not to be a passive role: inasmuch as women were to maintain society's moral standards, and therefore the morals of future generations, their social roles were of equal importance to those of the men, and they were to actively express and work to ensure their rights in this regard (Willard, 1889: 392-394).

It was this view of women and the family, not any antipathy to alcohol *per se,* that brought many women into the temperance ranks in the first place. Liquor, as they saw it, did more than bring personal hardship to individual women drinkers; it was also a direct threat to their children and husbands, and thus to their social status. It was this realization that enabled such diverse personalities as Frances Willard and other moderate drys to unite with zealots like Carry Nation on "Home Protection" (actually an official motto of the Woman's Christian Temperance Union) as one of the Temperance Movement's chief goals (Willard, 1889: 377-379). And it was in the home, they felt, that a woman could be most effective as a temperance worker; for there her opinions and concern for her loved ones could squarely confront the threat to the family. "Here woman bears sway," the reasoning of one dry speaker went, "and results for good or evil depend mainly upon her will." If women banished liquor from the home and worked for prohibition, she concluded, "we shall be safe; our children, our servants, our visitors will be safe," and the nation itself would be spared untold suffering (National Temperance Society, 1877: 185). If anything, then, temperance arguments like these served only to further entrench popular perceptions of woman's "proper" social role. The point here is, however, that whatever the context—that of the Temperance Movement or that of general attitudes—American gender roles were pretty clearly defined by the late nineteenth century.

PERCEPTIONS OF THE ALCOHOLIC

If Americans held some fairly uniform views on gender roles, at the same time they had also formed a consistent image of the alcoholic. The image was that of the now familiar picture of a Skid Row derelict, which was an established stereotype by the late 1800s. In fact it had matured in the popular view by at least the 1830s, and aspects of it can be traced back even further (Lender and Karn-chanapee, 1977). But in the post-Civil War years, with the rise of the view of the family exemplified in the "Home Protection" credo, the alcoholic stereotype took on a more threatening guise. For just as middle-class Americans saw the ideal woman as a paragon of social virtue and a guardian of the home, they saw the alcoholic as all that threatened her. Regardless of who alcoholics were in reality, or how they came to be alcoholics, the public saw them as men who either deserted, brutalized, or otherwise victimized their families. A constant concern of the champions of "Home Protection" was that a drunken husband could shatter the financial security and social prestige of his wife and family. "If he throws away his good name," one dry author warned, "she is compelled to share in all the disgrace and loss which follows so sad a prodigality" (Weld, 1851: 246). Worse, he said, was the fact that mothers often had to "shield . . . the child of inebriates; not only from the positive cruelty and injustice of such fathers," but also from neglect and "ill example" (Weld, 1851: 244; Smith, 1901: 192). There was, of course, an element of truth to all of this. One of the most tragic sides of alcoholism *is* the suffering of those close to the alcoholic, and stories of once-prosperous families dragged into poverty by drinking breadwinners were staples of the temperance literature between the 1830s and 1920s (Lender and Karnchanapee, 1977).

THE SPECIAL STIGMA

Gender obviously played a critical role in this alcoholic stereotype: in the popular view alcoholics were men, women were their victims. Everything the country believed generally about women on one hand, and about alcoholics on the other, left it unprepared to envision women with drinking problems as real women. Women were virtuous and pure, alcoholics were degraded; women defended the home, alcoholics imperiled it; and while mothers strove to raise their children in a moral environment, drunkards were constant impediments to the task. Thus, to be an alcoholic was to behave in a way that was so removed from public expectations of women in the nineteenth century that society could account for it only as a form of the most extreme deviance.

Popular reaction was such that it attached traits to its view of alcoholism in women that were absent or not as pronounced in the stereotype of the male alcoholic. Specifically, the popular mind linked alcoholism in women to sexual promiscuity and to the loss of motherly and family interests—both of which were anathema to the standards of the middle class. The first charge received particular credence. An intemperate woman's morals supposedly "deadened" under the influence of alcohol, one doctor wrote, and "no sacrifice . . . became too great for the gratification of the morbid appetite" (Crothers, 1878: 250). This in turn, as a range of sources from college presidents to temperance workers reported, led to the "ruin" of young women and to outright prostitution. Indeed, one of the WCTU's chief objections to the liquor traffic was its supposed ability to draw women into organized vice and white slavery (Stewart, 1899: 412; Griffin, 1960: 100; Dorchester, 1888: 444; Barker, 1905: 186; Davis, 1916: 60, 98). The connections drawn between alcohol and vice are in fact among the most graphic in the temperance literature: "I never saw a human being that loved liquor as she did," one writer claimed of a young prostitute. "At sixteen she was a confirmed drunkard and streetwalker. She was devoid of any moral principle and had a perfectly insane temper" (Shaw, 1910: 330). Nor was this sort of comment confined to temperance workers; for as the following case study from the *Quarterly Journal of Inebriety* illustrates, some of the most lurid associations of alcoholism with promiscuity and vice appeared in the medical literature (Mac-Nicholl, 1902: 334):

> Female, aged forty-nine, eldest child, brought up in luxury, educated in the best private schools and under the supervision of skilled governesses and a social environment suitable to her wealth and station. As a young child she gave evidence of subtle depravity. At fourteen she showed great moral perversion; at nineteen became a concert hall singer, a confirmed drunkard, a regular prostitute, and the mother of an illegitimate child by her own brother; at twenty-three a government marine was forced to marry her at the muzzle of a revolver. For years, she posed as a prize fighter in the various low dives of our larger cities. Five years prior to his death she was the acknowledged mistress of her own father. The illegitimate child, a female, lived with her great grandmother until six years of age, and was then taken by her own mother to live in a colored house of prostitution. For nine years this child was the victim of the most barbarous and revolting lechery, the mother profiting thereby.

And even one of the most scholarly investigations of alcohol problems of the period noted that some of the women who became impoverished through alcoholism, though not "common prostitutes," had nevertheless "led immoral lives" or were "unchaste" (Koren, 1916: 110-111). Alcoholism, then, as one temperance tract put it, was a likely sign that a woman had left "the paths of virtue . . . to spend a dreadful and pitiable life of sin" (Brown, 1873: 7). This same moral decline also allegedly led women away from their stations as protectors of the home. Intemperate women, a number of sources charged, became "negligent, imprudent, and irreflective," contributed to the impoverishment of their homes, and threatened to make American families "fountainheads of drunkenness" (Davis, 1916: 106; Koren, 1916: 110-111; Fish, 1872: 7). Worse, they abused or otherwise failed to care for their children. "When a woman drinks," one doctor warned, "she neglects her children, pawns their clothes, leaving them exposed to cold and disease, she neglects her home and her husband, driving him probably also to drink, and so leading to assault and perhaps murder" (Smith, 1901: 192). After the turn of the century, Commander Evangeline Booth (1928: 3, 9) of Salvation Army lamented the frequent reports from field workers of "babies killed through the unconscious actions of drunken parents," and tragedies such as a "newly born baby lying in the arms of a drink-soaked mother." Nor was this situation confined to the poor, for the WCTU charged that it existed in all classes. "It is by no means an unusual occurrence," complained one WCTU member, "to see middle-class ladies intoxicated in the streets and stores, sometimes with the pitiable addition to the scene of a little child, trying with manifest distress, to get the sick mamma to a place of safety" (National Temperance Society, 1877: 180).

The truth of these allegations was never fully the point; the real issue was the nature of the accusations, and the fact that in the eyes of society these were the worst indictments that anyone could bring against a woman. Viewed in this context, the special stigma against women alcoholics becomes fully understandable; both sexual misconduct and the neglect of the family struck directly at the sanctity of the home and thus at the social position and role of the ideal woman as defined by the social norms of the day. And the fact that these stereotypes of alcoholic behavior in women were generalizations drawn from just a few examples, or that they were equally true of men, did not lessen their impact on the women involved. Invariable, one doctor explained, Americans saw inebriate women as worse than drunken men anyway: "A debauched woman," he said, "is always, everywhere, a more terrible object to behold than a brutish man. We look to see women a little nearer to the angels" than men, "so their fall seems greater" (Day, 1867: 62). Under the circumstances, then, the rise of a stigma on women alcoholics during this historical period was perhaps unavoidable.

This special stigma, however, was such an obvious manifestation of an unfair double standard in social behavior that even a few staunch temperance advocates complained. "We deem women the weaker sex," noted one dry author, "yet we exact more of her than of man" (Weld, 1851: 245). A recovered male alcoholic, who by 1877 was a confirmed temperance advocate and anxious to help other drinkers, made a similar and revealing comment on the particular tragedy of the woman alcoholic (Doner, 1877: 19-20):

> Hopeless, indeed, seems the condition of fallen women. Men can reform; society welcomes them back to the path of virtue; a veil is cast over their conduct, and their vows of amendment are accepted and their promises to reform are hailed with great delight. But, alas! for poor women who have been tempted to sin by rum. For them there are no calls to come home; no sheltering arm; no acceptance of confessions and promises to amend. We may call them the hopeless class. For all others we have hope: The drunken man can throw down the filthy cup and reform; he can take his place again in society, and be welcomed back. But for the poor woman, after she once becomes debased by this fiery liquid, there seems to be no space for repentance; for her there is no hope and prayer. How seldom we attempt to reach and rescue her! For her there is no refuge.

Exceptions to this bleak outlook were rare in the contemporary literature. Women able to hide or overcome their problems with the help of families or private sanitariums stood a better chance of maintaining their social status than others. But in these circumstances their success in beating alcoholism rarely came before the public as examples of women who had triumphed over the bottle and, more important, as challenges to the view that women alcoholics inevitably became depraved and hopeless. Indeed, unless they had independent means or families to support them, the best that most intemperate women could hope for was help from charitable organizations in finding shelter and some kind of employment, or assistance in sobering up. But even when this was achieved, many observers doubted the ability of a recovered woman to remain abstinent or self-sufficient, much less socially acceptable. Commander Booth (1928: 10) told of one woman, formerly "without shame or decency who scrubbed only that she might drink." She became generally sober and learned to keep a neat apartment; but she was "not a strong character, and no matter how wistful in her desire to be a decent, respectable woman, she was helpless" in the face of alcohol and frequently relapsed. Another woman, who became abstinent after repeated drunkenness arrests, had the best wishes of the temperance workers who helped her reform, but not their confidence. "What the ultimate outcome will be," they said of her, "none can tell" (Shaw, 1910: 37). A few women also took advantage of temperance-sponsored work programs aimed at building abstinence. Such programs, however, reached relatively few, their results were modest, and they promised only a minimal working-class livelihood (Warren, 1851: 392-403). But even these tenuous recoveries from alcoholism were exceptions—so unusual that some contemporaries considered them nothing less than "evidence that there is no limit to the power and grace of God" (Shaw, 1910: 331).

HIDDEN ALCOHOLISM: THE CONSEQUENCES

Beyond the fairness of the matter, however, was the fact that the stigma against women was dangerous. Indeed, the prevailing wisdom of the late nineteenth and early twentieth centuries was that the physical impact of alcoholism was more damaging in women than in men. Most doctors who dealt with intemperate women were sure that this fact accounted for low recovery rates among their female patients. The superintendent of a woman's inebriate asylum, for instance, reported that relative to men, alcoholism advanced faster and was less curable in women (Crothers, 1878). Throughout the closing years of the nineteenth century comment in the *Quarterly Journal of Inebriety* consistently noted that women alcoholics were "more or less chronic" compared to men, and that for every recovered male there were "hundreds of women" beyond the hope of cure (Crothers, 1878: 248; Wilson, 1895: 254-255; Sparks, 1898: 315). Alcoholism was "bad enough" in men, another voice warned in an editorial (1899: 59), but in women it was even "more far-reaching and more dreadful in its results."

A study of the medical histories of alcoholics lends considerable credence to these observations. Horatio M. Pollock (1914), the statistician of the New York State Hospital Commission, analyzed the records of 1739 patients institutionalized for alcoholism between 1909 and 1912. He found that of the 1330 men under review, 586 (44%) had "recovered" before discharge, while only 118 (29%) of the 409 women regained their health. This was due, Pollock said, to a greater proportion of the women having more serious alcohol-related physical disorders: "as a class," he noted, they were "deteriorated to a greater degree than the men" (Pollock, 1914: 233). This fact was starkly evident from the medical records. Among the men, for example, the alcoholic condition found most often was acute hallucinosis (present in 39%), which was also one of the least physically damaging. The most frequent complication among women, however, was perhaps the worst—fully 35% of them presented with Korsakoff's Syndrome (as opposed to only 14% of the men), which, modern research has demonstrated, indicated longer and more destructive preadmission drinking careers (Pollock, 1914: 207; Keller and McCormick, 1968: 105, 122-123; Adams and Collins, 1971: 17, 33). In addition, only 11% of the men suffered from a nervous disability such as neuritis or polyneuritis, while Pollock's data noted these problems in over 32% of the women. Women also had slightly higher proportions of respiratory, digestive and genitourinary disorders, and more often had at least some kind of physical complication accompanying their alcoholism than men (59% versus 48%). Finally, the generally more serious health problems of the females made the death rate among them twice as high (15% versus 7%) as in the males (Pollock, 1914: 214-216, 235-236). Judging from this data, then, it is hard to disagree with Pollock's conclusion that, physically at least, alcoholism was most destructive in the institutionalized women.

Pollock's study, unfortunately was unique for the period, as analyses of different alcoholic populations were not nearly as comprehensive. But other evidence points subjectively to conclusions similar to his. Among the public inebriates arrested and sent to dry out at New York City's Bellevue Hospital in the 1880s, for instance, many of the women were in poorer health than the men. Specifically, the cases with "alcoholic paralysis (multiple neuritis)" were usually women (Dana, 1890: 265). Case studies reported by physicians in private and institutional practice also mentioned the relatively greater prevalence of multiple neuritis in women, as well as stressing their particularly violent reactions to delirium tremors (Staples, 1900: 414; Sanderson, 1902: 451-454). In this regard, the records of a Massachusetts asylum in the 1860s indicated that the institutionalized women alcoholics there may have been in worse overall condition than the men. Marginal notes denoting the severity of patient disorders were relatively more frequent for females, and were certainly graphic: one woman alcoholic was thought insane, while another "passed a terrible night, constantly screaming" (Fisher, 1861). Another report claimed that women alcoholics were going insane at twice the rate of their male counterparts (Smith, 1901: 193). And Dr. Agnes Sparks, perhaps the first woman physician to devote special attention to alcohol problems in other women, observed that their drinking patterns were less prone to induce periodic binges than a fairly steady consumption over a long span of time—which, if unnoticed and unchecked, could help explain the high incidence of Korsakoff cases reported by Pollock (Sparks, 1898: 33). While not as conclusive as Pollock's study, then, these other views easily contributed to the general opinion that the physical consequences of alcoholism were more pronounced in women than in men.

Contemporary theories varied on why alcohol problems took such different courses in the genders, although this was not from any lack of thought on the matter. Some inquiries focused on physiological distinctions between men and women, and on the nervous system of women in particular. Such thinking suggested that in regard to alcohol women were indeed the "weaker sex," as their nerves were supposedly more susceptible to the effects of alcohol. "There is no doubt," wrote Albert Day (1867: 63), who had specialized in treating alcoholics since the 1860s, "that the nervous system of woman is more exquisitely sensitive to suffering than that of a man," and that alcohol affected women accordingly. Writing in a similar vein, Dr. George Beard (1871: 138) claimed that compared to men, women were "relatively very frail," while an author in the *Quarterly Journal of Inebriety* noted in 1877 that the severity of alcoholism in women was due to their "peculiarly susceptible nervous organization" (Crothers, 1878: 247). But these observations were speculation, not based on research and never discussed in depth.

Indeed, most attention in this regard focused instead on what we now call "hidden alcoholism." While they never used the term, both lay and professional observers clearly described the process.

As one physician put it, because in American society it was "regarded as a great disgrace for" women "to be intemperate," they usually tried to conceal their drinking problems (Smith, 1901: 192; Crothers, 1878: 248). Alcoholism in women, another doctor noted, usually remained hidden a long time before (if ever) it came to medical attention, while still another practitioner lamented that whereas a male alcoholic "seldom attempts to deceive us," women generally did. "We need expect no help from her" in diagnosing the problem, he warned, as she often kept "the real cause of her suffering" a secret even from family and friends (Crothers, 1878: 248). In 1876, the president of the New York State WCTU claimed that many women, including "half the ladies of wealth and fashion," routinely "disguised" their alcohol problems. They allegedly accomplished the deception by constantly drinking small quantities of liquor, which kept them lightly but not visibly intoxicated, by using perfume to hide the smell of alcohol, and by inventing excuses to avoid company in order to "sleep it off" in private (Smith, 1901: 192; National Temperance Society, 1877: 179, 181). Families often assisted in shielding the woman alcoholic out of sympathy for her and out of fear that the entire household would be disgraced. And even when women sought or received help, there was still a premium placed on hiding the condition. Families sent wives and daughters to inebriate asylums quietly, with "few . . . suspecting the truth." At some institutions in the late nineteenth century, women received therapy in private rooms apart from the rest of the patients (National Temperance Society, 1877: 180-181; Clark, 1893: 82).

Clearly, then, the sexual double standard was already a major factor in hidden alcoholism among women at least a century ago. And considering that research has produced no other cause for the relatively severe health complications of women alcoholics in the past, it is not too much to assign most of the blame to the stigma born of the era's popular attitudes toward women and drinking.

CONCLUSION

There are, finally, a few things we can say in retrospect on the origins of this stigma on women alcoholics. It seems clear that, as much as anything else, women were victims of timing: if American attitudes on gender roles, as embodied in the prevalent views on the sanctity of the family, had not coincided with such a dark contemporary view of alcoholics, perhaps things could have been different. While it is possible that some other circumstances might also have raised special social sanctions against alcoholism in women (although we really have no way of knowing), as it was, the clash between views on the ideal woman and the popular stereotype of the alcoholic was too great. Women (and for that matter, anyone concerned with the nation's alcohol problems) were simply not free to deal with drinking as a distinct issue—which, in the context of the period, would have been tough enough anyway. They were forced as well to cope with the public's view that, as alcoholics, they were also pernicious threats to the moral and social standards of the entire nation. Their attempts to hide their drinking, and the medical consequences of these attempts, then, were hardly surprising; nor was it any accident that notice of hidden alcoholism among women first entered the medical literature (although, as we have noted, without the use of the term itself) in precisely this post-Civil war era.

There are implications in all of this for today. If the stigma grew as it did because of factors beyond drinking behavior alone—and even beyond the social sanctions brought against male alcoholics—it stands to reason that efforts to deal with alcohol problems in women today cannot be solely concerned with drinking either. For it is not just the familiar stigma against the alcoholic which women have contended with for over a century, but a stigma with roots deeply entrenched in attitudes toward what it means (and has meant) to be a woman in America. Perhaps it would be well to keep this historical legacy in view as society plans efforts to help women alcoholics today.

REFERENCES

Barker, J. M. *The Saloon Problem and Social Reform* (New York: Everett Press, 1905).

Beckman, L. J. "Women Alcoholics: A Review of Social and Psychological Studies," *Journal of Studies on Alcohol* 36 (1973): 797-824.

Beard, G. *Stimulants and Narcotics: Medically, Philosophically and Morally Considered* (New York: Putnam, 1871).

Booth, E. *Some Have Stopped Drinking* (Westerville, Ohio: American Issue Press, 1928).

Bordin, R. *Women and Temperance: The Quest for Power and Liberty, 1873-1900* (Philadelphia: Temple University Press, 1981).

Brown, G. *Lecture on Temperance: With Numerous Connundrums* (Paterson, N.J.: n.p., 1873).

Clark, C. S. *The Perfect Keeley Cure: Incidents at Dwight and "Through the Valley of the Shadow" into the Perfect Light* (Milwaukee: C. S. Clark, 1893).

Clark, N. *Deliver us From Evil: an Interpretation of American Prohibition* (New York: Norton, 1976).

Crothers, T. D. "Inebriety in Women," *Quarterly Journal of Inebriety,* 2 (1878): 247-250.

Dana, C. L. "A Study of Alcoholism as it Appears in the Bellevue Hospital Cells," *Quarterly Journal of Inebriety,* 12 (1890): 262-269.

Davis, E. S. (Comp.) *A Compendium of Temperance Truth* (Evanston, Ill.: National Woman's Christian Temperance Union, 1916).

Day, A. *Methomania: a Treatise on Alcohol Poisoning* (Boston: J. Campbell, 1867).

Doner, T. *Eleven Years a Drunkard: The Life of Thomas Doner* (Sycamore, Ill.: Doner, 1877).

Dorchester, D. *The Liquor Problem in all Ages* (New York: Phillips & Hunt, 1888).

Editorial. "Inebriety in Women," *Quarterly Journal of Inebriety,* 21 (1899): 59.

Epstein, B. *The Politics of Domesticity: Women, Evangelism, and Temperance in Nineteenth-Century America* (Middletown, Ct.: Wesleyan University Press, 1981).

Fish, H. C. *Drinking for Health: A Sermon* (New York: National Temperance Society Publication House, 1982).

Fisher Case Records. Cases Y-15, Y-53, Y-61 (Boston: Contway Library of Medicine, Harvard University, Rare Book Department, 1861-1862).

Garrett, G. R. & H. M. Bahr "Women on Skid Row," *Quarterly Journal of Studies on Alcohol* 34 (1973): 1228-1243.

Griffin, C. S. *Their Brothers' Keepers: Moral Stewardship in the United States, 1799-1865* (New Brunswick, N.J.: Rutgers U. Press, 1960).

Houghton, W. E. *The Victorian Frame of Mind* (New Haven: Yale U. Press, 1957).

Janeway, E. *Man's World, Woman's Place* (New York: Morrow, 1971).

Keller, M. & McCormick, M. *A Dictionary of Words About Alcohol* (New Brunswick, N.J.: Center of Alcohol Studies, 1968).

Koren, J. *Alcohol and Society* (New York: H. Holt, 1916).

Lender, M. E. "Women Alcoholics: Prevalence Estimates and their Problems as Reflected in Turn-of-the-Century Institutional Data," *International Journal of the Addictions* 16 (1981): 443-448.

Lender, M. E. & K. R. Karnchanapee "Temperance Tales: Antiliquor Fiction and American Attitudes Toward Alcoholics in the late 19th and early 20th Centuries," *Journal of Studies on Alcohol* 38 (1977): 1347-1370.

Lender, M. E. & J. K. Martin *Drinking in America: A History* (New York: Free Press, 1982).

Lisansky, E. S. "The Woman Alcoholic," *Annals of the American Academy of Political and Social Science* 315 (1958): 73-81.

MacNicholl, T. A. "Alcohol a Cause of Degeneracy," *Quarterly Journal of Inebriety* 24 (1902): 330-335.

Mulford, H. A. "Women and Men Problem Drinkers: Sex Differences in Patients Served by Iowa's Community Alcoholism Centers," *Journal of Studies on Alcohol* 38 (1977): 417-430.

National Temperance Society *Centennial Temperance Volume: A Memorial of the International Temperance Conference, Held in Philadelphia, June, 1876* (New York: National Temperance Society and Publication House, 1877).

Pollock, H. M. "A Statistical Study of 1,739 Patients With Alcoholic Psychoses," *State Hospital Bulletin* 7 (1914): 204-268.

Sanderson, H. E. "Alcoholic Psychoses in Women," *Quarterly Journal of Inebriety* 24 (1902): 452-458.

Shaw, E. R. (ed.) *The Curse of Drink: or Hell's Commerce* (Grand Rapids, MI.: n.p., 1960).

Smith, H. "Alcohol in Relation to Women," *Quarterly Journal of Inebriety* 23 (1901): 190-193.

Sparks, A. "Alcoholism in Women: Its Cause, Consequence, and Cure," *Quarterly Journal of Inebriety* 20 (1898): 31-37.

Staples, H. L. "Alcoholism," *Quarterly Journal of Inebriety* 22 (1900): 412-425.

Stewart, E. D. *Memories of the Crusade* (Columbus, Oh.: Hubbard, 1889).

Victor, M., Adams, R. D. & Collins, G. H. *The Wernicke-Korsakoff Syndrome: a Clinical and Pathological Study of 245 Patients, 82 with Post-mortem Examinations* (Philadelphia: F. A. Davis, 1971).

Warren, C. J. "The Industrial Temperance Home," *National Temperance Magazine* 1 (1851): 392-403.

Weld, H. H. "Women and Temperance," *American Temperance Magazine* 2 (1851): 243-254.

Willard, F. E. *Glimpses of Fifty Years: The Autobiography of an American Woman* (Chicago: Woman's Temperance Publishing Association, 1889).

Wilson, A. "Inebriety in Women," *Quarterly Journal of Inebriety* 17 (1895): 254-256.

The Summer School of Alcohol Studies: An Historical and Interpretive Review

Gail Gleason Milgram, Ed.D.

INTRODUCTION

This essay on the Summer School of Alcohol Studies begins somewhat earlier than its founding in 1943 by the Section of Studies on Alcohol of the Laboratory of Applied Physiology at Yale University. The earlier beginning was selected to provide a perspective and context in which to view the School. The Summer School of Alcohol Studies and the changes which occurred through its history (e.g., time frame, format, content, student population, etc.) are presented; some of the significant happenings in the alcohol studies field are also interjected into the historical review. In this way, it is hoped that the School can be viewed as the growing and changing institution that it is and its impact on the alcohol studies field can be evaluated.

The Summer School of Alcohol Studies perhaps more than any institution in the alcohol studies field, demonstrates our interconnectedness. E. M. Jellinek, Bill W., Marty Mann, Mark Keller, Selden Bacon and many others of significance in the alcohol field were discussing, debating and learning from each other at one point in time. The Summer School enabled them to share their knowledge with others.

SUMMER SCHOOL OF ALCOHOL STUDIES

After thirteen years of Prohibition, the Constitution was amended and Prohibition was abolished in 1933. Though many of the people of the U.S.A. were relieved that alcohol was again legal, most also

Gail Gleason Milgram, Professor/Executive Director of the Summer School of Alcohol Studies, Center of Alcohol Studies, Rutgers University.

had high hopes that Prohibition had eliminated the problem of alco-holism. However, Mark Keller notes that approximately 10,000 al-coholics were admitted to one hospital in New York City in 1933 (Keller, 1979).

At about the same time, the fellowship of Alcoholics Anonymous was founded by Dr. Bob and Bill W. in Akron, Ohio (1935); by 1939 the membership of A.A. had reached 100. The phenomenal growth of this fellowship is more clearly perceived by the 1941 membership; the number in A.A. in early 1941 was approximately 2,000. By the end of the year, the total was approximately 8,000. The year 1941 also marked the founding of the Allied Liquor Indus-tries. This group changed its name in 1946 to Licensed Beverage In-dustries and in 1973 to the Distilled Spirits Council of the United States (DISCUS).

Dr. Norman Jolliffe, Chief of Medical Services of the Psychiatric Division of Bellevue Hospital in New York City in the mid-1930s, was treating individuals with illnesses related to alcoholism and con-cluded that alcoholism, rather than the medical disorders that were associated with it, should be studied. In 1935, a research project was designed; Jolliffe felt that the study should incorporate the work of physicians, psychiatrists, psychologists, public health nurses, psy-chiatric social workers, social scientists and anthropologists.

Dr. Howard W. Haggard was a member of the scientific advisory committee formed by Jolliffe; Dr. Haggard was the Director of the Laboratory of Applied Physiology at Yale University, which was al-ready conducting research on the metabolism of alcohol and its ef-fects. This research had begun prior to Dr. Haggard's appointment as Director; Professor Yandell Henderson, who was also a member of the scientific advisory committee had been the founder and Direc-tor of the Laboratory of Applied Physiology. Henderson's work focused on the nature of human intoxication. The Research Council on Problems of Alcohol evolved out of the scientific advisory com-mittee founded by Jolliffe; the aim of the Research Council was to seek financial support for research on alcohol problems.

A review of the biological literature on alcohol was the first grant received by the Council. E. M. Jellinek was hired as the project director and offices were set up in the New York Academy of Medicine. The staff was "a multidisciplinary team representing clinical and experimental medicine, physiology, both clinical and experimental psychology, both the psychologically and physiologically oriented branches of psychiatry, biometrics, and documentation'' (Keller, 1979).

When the review was finished, though not fully written, the grant money was exhausted. Howard W. Haggard invited E. M. Jellinek to Yale to complete the writing of the review. Others of the original team (Dr. Giorgio Lolli, Dr. Martin Gross, Dr. Anne Roe, Mark Keller and Vera Efron) joined Jellinek and new staff (Dr. Seldon Bacon, a sociologist and Dr. Edward G. Baird, a jurisprudent) were added. This interdisciplinary group formed the Section of Studies on Alcohol with Jellinek as its first director. The Section on the Studies on Alcohol later changed its name to the Center of Alcohol Studies. Upon completion of the review, Howard W. Haggard founded the *Quarterly Journal of Studies on Alcohol* in 1940. In the first two volumes of this interdisciplinary periodical (1940-41 and 1941-42), the review papers were published.

Research, education, treatment and prevention were the founding cornerstones of the Center of Alcohol Studies. In light of these four major goals, the Center founded the Yale Plan Clinics, the first public outpatient alcoholism clinics for the treatment of alcoholism. Multidisciplinary teams using a variety of techniques treated alcoholics; research on alcoholism treatment was a viable part of this program. The Center also initiated an industry program for treating employed alcoholics. Dr. Anne Roe of the Center conducted a review of existing school education materials; the Center also helped to form an organization of educators, the American Association for Instruction on Alcohol and Narcotics, to stimulate changes in education about alcohol in the schools.

A National Committee for Education on Alcoholism was founded at the Summer School of Alcohol Studies in 1944 by Mrs. Marty Mann with the help of some of the Center's faculty and sponsored by the Center. This committee was supported in its early years by the Center and maintained its headquarters at the Yale Center of Alcohol Studies for its first five years. The goal established for the committee was ''to bring to all America the message that alcoholism is an illness which can be banished by definite therapeutic means''; the aims were scientific, practical, educational, and humanitarian. In the first four years of the National Committee's existence, forty-one local committees were formed in cities throughout the United States. Mrs. Marty Mann was the Executive Director, the Board of Directors included Selden D. Bacon, Howard W. Haggard, M.D.

and E. M. Jellinek. The Advisory Board consisted of thirty-three people; Bill W., Mary Pickford, Karl A. Menninger, M.D., Harry M. Trebout, M.D., and Charles Jackson were members of the Advisory Board. The National Committee for Education on Alcoholism is now known as the National Council on Alcoholism.

It was felt by Center faculty that "the prevention of inebriety through civic activities is seriously hampered by the lack of a sufficiently large number of persons who have a broad and scientific understanding of the problems of alcohol and who could qualify as leaders in their communities. Education of such leaders seems to be essential in preparing the way for the prevention of inebriety" (Current Notes, 1943). To meet this need, the Center founded the first Summer School of Alcohol Studies in 1943 where all disciplines and professions, including Alcoholics Anonymous, could educate future researchers, educators and community leaders.

The first Summer School of Alcohol Studies was held at Yale University in 1943. The School, directed by E. M. Jellinek, Sc.D., lasted for six weeks and admitted school teachers and administrators, ministers and religious workers of all denominations, welfare workers, probation officers, and others engaged in activities in which a knowledge of alcohol problems would be advantageous. Though the School had no outside sponsorship, cooperation of religious and educational bodies was obtained. The National Education Association provided scholarships to educators and the Commission on Religion and Health provided scholarships to clergy and religious workers. Financial assistance to other professional workers, (e.g., welfare workers, public officials, etc.) was provided by the School. "To render the findings of scientific research available for application to the actual problems of alcohol in the community" was the object of the School (Summer School brochure, 1943). The aim was to provide a thorough grounding in all the problems of alcohol.

To accomplish this the eight main courses of study in the 1943 School included the following: introduction, physiological aspects, alcohol and traffic, personality and constitution, statistics, social measures, legislative control, and prevention and treatment of alcoholics. There were also three seminar subjects and three public lectures totaling 164 hours (102 hours of lectures, and 62 hours of seminars).

The lecturers strongly represented the medical profession (8), others, the legal profession (2), anthropology (2), applied physiology (2), statistics (2). Bill W., the co-founder of Alcoholics

Anonymous, also lectured, as did E. M. Jellinek, the School's director.

In 1944, the United States Public Health Service labeled alcoholism the nation's fourth largest public health problem. This generated enthusiasm in the field of alcohol studies and expanded the student enrollment in the Summer School. One of the students in the 1944 School was Mrs. Marty Mann, who in 1944, following the Summer School, was a founder of the National Committee for Education on Alcoholism. The 1944 School changed the time format to four weeks, added an Assistant Director, Rev. Francis McPeel, and continued the format of daily lectures, seminars and discussion periods. The group of lecturers expanded to thirty, including seven physicians, five lawyers, three members of the clergy, and three individuals representing applied physiology. There were also lecturers from social work (3), psychology (2), sociology (2), criminal psychopathology (1), economics (1), traffic and transportation (1), and education (1). Alcoholics Anonymous was also represented by Bill W. The population for admissions and scholarships remained the same as in 1943.

In 1945, the lecture topics were grouped under seven headings: introduction, effects of alcohol on the individual and on society, use of alcoholic beverages, prevention of inebriety, measures of control, and treatment. Seminars were conducted on mobilization of community resources, the alcohol problem and the church, legal control, alcohol education and therapy of alcoholism. Mrs. Marty Mann joined the lecturers in the 1945 School. The 1946 School was similar in format and faculty to that described for 1945, except for the addition of one representative of the distilled spirits industry as a lecturer. The student population and scholarship support also remained constant.

The School's format changed in 1947; the first two weeks contained general lectures which focused on effects and use of alcohol, psychological factors related to alcoholism, the magnitude of the problem, formal controls, and treatment. The third and fourth weeks increased the seminar offerings to six by the addition of a research seminar. The faculty of thirty-seven were composed of the disciplines noted for other years plus the National President of the Women's Christian Temperance Union and two representatives of the distilled spirits industry.

In 1948, physicians and psychologists were added to the student population. The first two weeks of general lectures followed the pattern of other years; however, the third and fourth weeks offered two separate curricula:

1. Curricula A for educators, those interested in legal controls, and related subjects;
2. Curricula B for physicians, social workers, and others interested primarily in care and treatment of alcoholics.

The faculty in 1948 included a representative of the U.S. Brewers Foundation and the Maryland Anti-Saloon League. The scholarship support in the 1948 School was maintained from the National Education Association, the Commission on Religion and Health and the School.

Two sessions of the Summer School were conducted in 1949: an Eastern session of four weeks duration and a Western session of three weeks time. The Eastern session was housed at Yale University as in previous years and the Western session was located at Trinity University in San Antonio, Texas. The School's tuition identified two separate categories of participants. Category I included ministers, physicians, social and welfare workers, probation and parole officers, teachers, nurses, graduate students, and federal, state and municipal employees. The tuition for this category was approximately half the cost of the tuition for Category II, which consisted of all students not specified in the first group.

Nineteen hundred and forty-nine marks the founding year for the Addiction Research Foundation in Canada and the National States Conference on Alcholism, which was renamed in 1956 as the North American Association of Alcoholism Programs and in 1972, the Alcohol and Drug Problems Association.

Al-Anon, the fellowship for spouses and significant others in the life of an alcoholic, was founded in 1951. The acknowledgement of the impact of alcoholism on family members and the availability of help for these individuals was clearly identified by the founding of Al-Anon. The year 1951 also marked the founding of the North Conway Institute by Rev. David Works. The goal of the Institute was, and is, to encourage church groups to develop active ministries to alcoholics. It also identified as a role of the church, the fostering of public awareness of alcohol-related problems.

The 1951 Yale University SSAS was directed by Selden D. Bacon, Ph.D., who was to remain as SSAS director through 1962. Though the student body's composition was similar to previous years, the availability of scholarship support had changed. The application and awarding of scholarships was through the School. This practice was maintained until 1958.

A geographic distribution of the 1,168 students who had attended the School from 1943-1950 showed representation from 47 states of the United States and the District of Columbia, from nine provinces of Canada and from nine other countries. A review of the professional/occupational affiliation of the students identified a constant rise in the proportion of students with professional background; a decrease in the number of clergy (once more than a third of the student body, comprised less than a fifth in 1950); the proportion of professional temperance workers had dropped markedly; educators represented the largest single group in the student body (representing health and physical education departments of high schools and colleges and state departments of education); and physicians, psychologists, and persons in various phases of rehabilitation work had formed a steadily increasing proportion of the student body.

In 1953, the School expanded its objectives to meet the needs of professional and nonprofessional people. The lectures were organized around the following topical areas: social problems, personality development theories, problems of alcohol, physiological and psychological effects of alcohol, and the nature and treatment of alcoholism. During the third and fourth weeks, afternoons were devoted to seminars in education, the role of the church, rehabilitation, medical therapy and health organization.

A one-week Industrial Institute was conducted in 1953 during the Summer School. This session was open to representatives of business, industry and labor who were engaged in industrial health, personnel work, industrial relations or related activity. The purpose of the Institute was to acquaint selected representatives of business and industry with the nature of problem drinking in industry, policies of treatment, procedures and resources for treatment, and programs of education and prevention.

SSAS 1954 included afternoon seminars in the second week and added the topics of nursing, community organization, social work and special studies. A three-day Nurses Institute on Alcoholism followed the 1954 School. Afternoon seminars during SSAS 1955 were offered in education, ministry, community health and therapy. The therapy seminar was further delineated into four sections for physicians, social workers, nurses and psychologists and rehabilitation workers. A one-week Refresher Session, open to graduates of the School from 1943-1955, followed the 1955 School.

Leon A. Greenberg, Ph.D. became the Director of the Laboratory of Applied Physiology in 1957; 1957 was an important year for the alcohol field as it was the year Alateen was founded and E. M. Jellinek began a study of attitudes throughout the world toward the concept of alcoholism as a disease. This project was funded by the Christopher D. Smithers Foundation and resulted in the publication of Jellinek's *Disease Concept of Alcoholism* in 1960. In this text, Jellinek explored the historical development of attitudes toward alcoholism as a disease; analyzed the varied scientific approaches to the problem; and, finally, reviewed beliefs and attitudes in different segments of the public in countries around the world (Jellinek, 1960).

The only area of change in the 1958 School was mention of scholarship availability through state or provincial commissions on alcoholism and denominational affiliations; this pattern of external support continued through the 1966 School. Two seminar topics were also added in 1958: enforcement and corrections and rehabilitation. The American Medical Association recognized alcoholism as a disease in 1958; this recognition was a necessary and vital element for the scientific growth of the alcohol studies field and for public attitudes and support. A public health seminar was added to the School in 1959 and an Industry Seminar added in 1960. In other aspects the School remained the same as in previous years; 1961 continued the pattern.

The Cooperative Commission on the Study of Alcoholism was established in 1961 and financed by a grant from the National Institute of Mental Health. The membership of the Commission, directed by Dr. R. Nevitt, was drawn from a variety of professionals and scientific disciplines. *Alcohol Problems: A Report to the Nation, by the Cooperative Commission on the Study of Alcoholism* was prepared by Thomas F. A. Plaut, Ph.D. and published in 1967. The report's four main areas included societal disagreement about alcohol use, treatment and management of problem drinking and a coordinated national policy toward alcohol problems. Collaborative efforts of scientists, professional workers, legislators, government officials, citizens and other organizations were called on by the Commission to deal with the problems associated with the use of alcohol. The Commission concluded its work and was disbanded in 1966.

The year 1962 marked significant changes for the Center and SSAS. The Center of Alcohol Studies moved to Rutgers University; this move was made possible by financial support from the National Institute of Mental Health and the Christopher D. Smithers Foundation (founded in 1952) of New York. Selden D. Bacon, Ph.D., became the Director of the Center in 1962 and Raymond McCarthy, A.M., Ed.M., became the Executive Director of the Summer School.

The School's admission requirements in 1963 listed the following criteria: professionally qualified applicants who have major responsibility for work in field of alcoholism/alcohol problems; or others with college education or equivalent experience.

The Summer School of Alcohol Studies became a three-week School in 1964, the time frame which is still in effect. This year also clearly indicated the School's role in providing intensive, specialized training to professionals or persons with experience in the field. The format of the School changed significantly to support the aim of specialized training. Each student was to enroll in two specialized courses: one for an evaluation and grade and the other one on an audit basis. This system was maintained until SSAS 1975 when both courses were taken for an evaluation. Thirteen courses in 1964 focused on the social implications of alcohol use in American society; alcoholism services; counseling in alcoholism; public health and voluntary agency resources; the role of labor-management; services and programs for alcoholic patients and their families; institutional programs for homeless alcoholics; pastoral counseling and drinking and driving.

A two-week Physicians Institute held concurrently with the Summer School of Alcohol Studies, began in 1964 and continued through 1969. This program was designed for physicians who wished to be informed about current research knowledge and clinical practice in alcoholism; it was open to holders of medical degrees and medical students by arrangement. A course for physicians, "Medical Aspects of Alcoholism" was added to SSAS in 1970.

The Northeast Institute, a one-week Institute co-sponsored by the State Alcoholism programs of nine northeastern states, also began in 1964 and continued through 1969. Providing a general overview of problems of alcohol and alcoholism for board members of official and voluntary agencies, civic leaders and officers, and others lacking experience in the field, this Institute also ran concurrently with the Summer School. Milton A. Maxwell, Ph.D., became the School's Director in 1965. Nursing was added in 1965 and three new courses were added in 1967: Group Dynamics in Alcoholism Programming, Alcoholics and Vocational Rehabilitation, and Drinking and Law Enforcement. Kemper scholarships for teachers in schools of nursing were added to the School in 1967 and maintained through the 1979 School. U.S.P.H.S. traineeships for public health workers were available from 1967 to 1970. Drinking and Law Enforcement was deleted in 1968 and Problems of Drinking and Driving was added. This course was deleted from the offerings in 1970 and three courses were added: Medical Aspects of Alcoholism (the course for physicians mentioned earlier); The Clergyman, The Community and Alcohol Problems; and Law Enforcement and Alcohol Problems. The Smithers Fellowships for attorneys and law students were added in 1970. The Alumni Association of the Summer School of Alcohol Studies also began providing scholarship awards in the early 1970s.

Also in 1970, Congress passed the Comprehensive Alcohol Abuse and Alcohol Prevention Treatment, and Rehabilitation Act. This act established the National Institute on Alcohol Abuse and Alcoholism to direct efforts against alcoholism at the federal level. "The new unit—the National Institute on Alcohol Abuse and Alcoholism—gave the alcoholism constituency a seemingly permanent voice in public health program and planning" (Lender, 1982). The Uniform Alcoholism and Intoxication Act of 1971, enacted by many states in the 1970s, substituted medical treatment for alcoholism for many alcohol related legal infractions that previously were handled by the criminal justice system.

Program Evaluation and Research was added to the course list in 1972, making the total of course offerings 19 for 1972 and 1973. The A. E. Bennett scholarships for physicians were offered for the first time in 1972; these were maintained through 1981. A triennial refresher course (five-day) for alumni was held in 1972. Ronald Lester, M.P.H., became the School's Director 1974-1982. Alcoholism and Public Health Nursing was deleted in 1974; however, The Older Person and Alcohol Use and Understanding and Working with A.A. were added to the course offerings bringing the total to twenty.

John A. Carpenter, Ph.D., became the Center's Director in 1975, following Selden Bacon's retirement. The *Quarterly Journal of Studies on Alcohol* became the *Journal of Studies on Alcohol.* SSAS added two courses in 1975: Program Administration and Management and Multiple Drug Usage in America: Problems and Perspectives. Multiple Drug Usage was the first Summer School offering to focus on drugs other than alcohol. The refresher course for alumni was conducted in 1976; this five-day program focused on preventive strategies, primary prevention, and education and mass persuasion in the reduction of alcohol problems.

SSAS 1976 deleted Law Enforcement and Alcohol Problems from the course offerings and added six new courses: Philosophical Bases of Preventing Alcohol Problems, Program Development and Grantsmanship, Alcoholism and Criminal Justice, Alcoholism and Women, Alcohol and Blacks, and Alcohol and Highway Safety. The Smithers Fellowships were deleted from the sources of scholarship support in 1976. Scholarships to the School were available to educators from a new source of support in 1976, the Prudential Insurance Company of America, Inc.; these scholarship awards have continued through the present day.

The New Jersey Summer School of Alcohol and Drug Abuse Studies was founded in 1976 to meet the education and training needs of the state and surrounding area and in so doing fill the void created when the Northeast Institute (a similar concept and program) ended in 1969. This one-week endeavor, which is still in operation, is sponsored by the Center of Alcohol Studies and the Divisions of Alcoholism and Narcotic and Drug Abuse of the New Jersey State Department of Health. It is also co-sponsored by the Prudential Insurance Company of America, Inc. Specialized courses, general lectures and special interest seminars are offered during the New Jersey School.

SSAS 1977 and 1978 maintained the same format and courses (total of 27) as in 1976. The one-week Alumni Institute of 1978 focused on alcohol and sexuality; the Alumni Association voted in 1978 to have institutes occur every two years rather than the traditional three years. Though the course offerings in the 1979 School totaled 29, there were three deletions: Organizing and Developing Alcoholism Programs in Public Health Settings, Philosophical Bases of Programs, and Pastoral Counseling with Alcoholics. Current Problems, Policies and Issues; Medical Implications of Alcoholism; Preventing Substance Abuse; Counseling Children of Alcoholics; and Sexuality Issues in Counseling were the five new courses.

Alcohol and Highway Safety and Sexuality Issues in Counseling were deleted in the 1980 School and Social Impact of Alcoholism was added, bringing the total course offerings of the School to twenty-eight. The Distilled Spirits Council of the United States (DISCUS) began providing scholarships to SSAS in 1980. The Alumni Institute, held in 1980, focused on alcohol and other drugs.

The total of twenty-eight courses was maintained in 1981 though Function and Structure of Alcoholism Services; The Homeless, Non-Family Alcoholic; and Social Impact of Alcoholism were deleted. Motivational Counseling in Alcoholism; Issues in the Treatment of Alcoholism and Counseling the Gay Alcoholic were added.

Gail Gleason Milgram, Ed.D. became the School's Executive Director in 1982. SSAS 1982 offered twenty-nine courses though many offerings had been deleted and others added. The course additions included: Fund Raising in the Private Sector; Health Care Management of the Alcoholic; Alcoholism and the Hispanic Population; Sexuality, Alcohol and Family Intimacy; and Diet Therapy in Prevention and Treatment of Substance Abuse. An Alumni Institute was held in 1982; Alcohol, Sexuality, and Personal Growth was the Institute's topic.

Nineteen hundred eighty-three marked a year of growth for the Center of Alcohol Studies and the Summer School of Alcohol Studies; the School's course offerings expanded to thirty-four. Peter E. Nathan, Ph.D., became the Director of the Center and has added a clinical component again to the Center's mission. The Center had founded the Yale Plan Clinics and the present addition of the clinical division returns one of the original major goals of the Center. The 1984 Summer School of Alcohol Studies is the forty-second annual session. The emphasis is on the forty specialized courses, supported and supplemented by a strong program of general lectures and special interest seminars. Students register for two courses; each course meets formally for eighty minutes each morning for a total of twenty hours. The courses can be viewed in major categories: counseling courses, courses dealing with special populations, societal aspects, other drugs, legal aspects, sexuality, and medical aspects and health. The others cover A.A., the church, prevention, community, supervision, diet, program management, and grant/proposal writing. General lectures and special interest seminars support the course offerings.

The course instructors represent major disciplines as in previous years; medical and health care professionals, psychologists, sociologists, social workers, lawyers, educators, health specialists, clergy, and a nutritionist make up the faculty. These individuals are from treatment facilities, academic institutions, national programs, state alcoholism agencies, industry, and private practice.

Approximately 12,000 students have attended the School since its inception in 1943. They have come from each of the fifty states, the ten Canadian provinces, and four other countries. A wide range of backgrounds, experience, and interests has characterized the population. A brief review of the statistics on the student population of the last five years of the School highlights some general information and indicates some trends. The sex ratio has somewhat changed; males represented the majority of the students in the years from 1977 through 1979—approximately 54%, whereas females were 54% of the population in 1982. In terms of age, the ranges of 18-24 and over 64 represent the smallest portion of the population (approximately 5%); and 7% are in the age range of 55-64.

The percentage of individuals who indicate membership in the fellowship of Alcoholics Anonymous has increased in recent years: in the years 1977-1979, 43% indicated A.A. membership; in 1982, 49% noted their A.A. affiliation. Since Al-Anon membership was not asked on the anonymous evaluation instrument prior to 1980, it is not possible to view change. However, approximately 20% of the population in 1982 identified affiliation with Al-Anon. There is a definite trend in the level of educational sophistication of the participants. In 1977, 13.9% had received a B.S., 22.7% a master's degree, and 4.4% a doctorate. In 1982, 24.4% had a B.S. degree, 28.7% a master's degree, and 7.2% a doctorate. Also, approximately 34% of the population had attended another school of alcohol or drug studies of at least a week's duration prior to attendance at SSAS.

Primary work areas of responsibility also indicate some changes. Counselors made up approximately 43% of the population in 1977-1978, and 60% in 1982; administrators comprised 23% of the group in 1977-1978 and 13% in 1982. Educators represented approximately 5% of the student body five years ago and 10% of the group in 1982. The nursing population of approximately 5% has remained somewhat constant.

DISCUSSION

Prior to the 1920s, the alcoholic (called "the drunkard" during this time) was viewed as a moral degenerate. The popular view in the U.S.A. was that drunkenness could be eliminated if alcohol was unavailable. During the thirteen year period of Prohibition, the term alcoholism replaced drunkenness. This is not to imply that alcohol was totally unavailable, but rather to imply a softening of attitudes toward individuals who were experiencing alcohol problems.

The 1930s experienced Repeal (1933) and left the country with ambivalent attitudes toward alcohol. The "wet" vs "dry" thinking was still very much present and led to vague ways of handling the official reintroduction of alcohol into society. During the same period, Alcoholics Anonymous was founded and studies of alcoholism were stimulated.

The 1940s witnessed significant growth in what was to become the alcohol studies field. The Yale Center of Alcohol Studies was founded and the Summer School of Alcohol Studies began; the National Council on Alcoholism has its beginning at the Summer School and Center of Alcohol Studies. Alcoholism was also labelled a disease by the U.S. Department of Health in this time period.

The School itself began with 23 lecturers of various disciplines and about seventy students. School teachers and administrators, ministers and religious workers, and probation workers made up the student body. As the School evolved through the forties, the time frame changed from six weeks to four weeks and the student population increased and included physicians, social workers, welfare workers, nurses and federal, state and municipal workers. By 1949, psychologists and persons in rehabilitation work were also in attendance.

Al-Anon, the North Conway Institute, and Alateen were founded in the 1950s. Jellinek's disease concept of alcoholism was formulated and the American Medical Association recognized alcoholism as a disease (1958). The Summer School offered afternoon seminars and periodically provided separate tracts of shorter duration for industry, nurses and alumni.

The Cooperative Commission on the Study of Alcoholism was formed in 1960 and the Commission's report, published in 1967, highlighted the disagreement about alcohol use that was still prevalent in the country and called for a national policy to address alcohol problems. The Center of Alcohol Studies moved to Rutgers University in the 1960s, as did the Summer School of Alcohol Studies. The School's time frame changed to the three-week format which is still present today. Professionally qualified applicants who have major responsibility for work in the alcohol field made up the student body. To meet the needs of the participants and also the field of alcohol studies, specialized training via thirteen courses was introduced by the School. A two-week Physicians Institute ran concurrently with the School and a separate one-week Northeast Institute was designed to meet the need for introductory training in the region.

The 1970s were significant in two areas in the alcohol field: The National Institute on Alcohol Abuse and Alcoholism (NIAAA) was founded to direct efforts against alcoholism at the federal level and the Uniform Alcoholism and Intoxication Act substituted medical treatment for many alcohol-related infractions that had previously been handled by the criminal justice system. Alcoholism research and literature also expanded.

The Summer School of Alcohol Studies also grew during the 1970s. The course offerings had expanded to almost thirty; courses for counselors had increased considerably as did the courses directed toward special populations (e.g., adolescents, women, Blacks). [Two courses were taken for evaluation and credit, indicating the strong trend for specialized content.] The student population reached its largest size of five-hundred individuals from across the U.S.A. and many foreign countries.

A growing need for basic introductory training in the alcohol studies field was again apparent in the 1970s. The one-week New Jersey Summer School of Alcohol and Drug Studies was designed to meet this need. The New Jersey School expanded to approximately two-hundred students in the 1970s and received students from a larger geographic area in each succeeding year. The expanding trend of the New Jersey School continued in the 1980s; approximately two-hundred and fifty students presently attend each School. The School has maintained its original mission to provide basic training to those new to the field and has also added advanced courses to meet the need of the individual in the field for additional training.

The Summer School of Alcohol Studies has continued to grow in the 1980s. The course offerings have expanded to forty (1984) to meet the needs of the diverse student body; a student body which has become increasingly more sophisticated as the field has grown over the years; the educational level of participants rises every year and the number of individuals who have had prior training in the alcohol studies field also increases yearly. Counselors represent the largest single part (60%) of the student population. Interestingly, this population was not even mentioned on the brochures in the early days of the School.

BIBLIOGRAPHY

Alcoholics Anonymous World Services, Inc. *Alcoholics Anonymous Comes of Age: A Brief History of A.A.* New York: Alcoholics Anonymous World Services, Inc., 1957.

Anderson, D. "Alcohol and Public Opinion" *Quarterly Journal of Studies on Alcohol*, (3), 1942.

Cooperative Commission on the Study of Alcoholism. Alcohol Problems: A Report to the Nation (prepared by Thomas F. A. Plaut, Ph.D.) Oxford University Press, NY: Coop. Comm., 1967.

"Current Notes: Summer School of Alcohol Studies, Yale University," *Quarterly Journal of Studies on Alcohol*, Vol. 3, 1943.

Ewing, J. A. and Rouse, B. A. (Ed.) *Drinking: Alcohol in American Society-Issues and Current Research.* Chicago: Nelson-Hall, 1978.

"Farewell Yale . . . and Rutgers, Hail!" A note on the Transit of the Quarterly Journal of Studies on Alcohol. *Quarterly Journal of Studies on Alcohol*, Vol. 23, No. 1, 1962.

Jellinek, E. M. *The Disease Concept of Alcoholism*, New Haven, Ct.; College and University Press, 1960.

Keller, M. "Mark Keller's History of the Alcohol Field." *The Drinking and Drug Practices Surveyor*, Number 14, March 1979.

Keller, M. "Multidisciplinary Perspectives on Alcoholism and the Need for Integration." *Journal of Studies on Alcohol*, Vol. 36, No. 1, 1975.

Lender, M. E. and Martin, J. K. *Drinking in America: A History.* New York: The Free Press; A Division of Macmillan Publishing Co., Inc., 1982.

Page, P. B., Archives and Manuscripts: An Inventory (1789-1981). New Brunswick, New Jersey: Rutgers Center of Alcohol Studies, 1982.

Summer School of Alcohol Studies, Brochures from 1943 through 1983. New Haven, Ct., Yale University and New Brunswick, NJ: Rutgers Center of Alcohol Studies.

Thinking About Drinking. New Brunswick, NJ. Rutgers Center of Alcohol Studies. (Note: No date on pamphlet.)

Alcoholism Rehabilitation: Getting Involved— A Memoir of the 60s

Sheila B. Blume, M.D.

My involvement in alcoholism treatment began during my first week of psychiatric training, at a large state hospital in New York. Like most other first year psychiatric residents, I had often encountered alcoholic people during my medical education, but had never been taught to confront their alcoholism. In Boston, where I went to medical school, many of the patients from whom we learned were alcoholics, yet that fact was generally accepted as an immutable personal characteristic rather than an illness requiring treatment.[1] Case histories often began "This 57 year old alcoholic white male entered the hospital because of . . ." It was like saying the patient was Jewish or Panamanian, merely a descriptive term. It was quite different from using the term "diabetic", for instance, which called for a medical assessment of diet, blood sugar, adequacy of control of the disease, etc. The only direct teaching I can recall on the subject was a few minutes during a psychoanalytic lecture on oral traits. My clinical psychiatric experience had consisted of talking for a few supervised hours with a schizophrenic patient who had undergone lobotomy. This was not atypical of medical education in the '50s.

Along with the lack of information about alcoholism came a transmission of attitudes which were uniformly negative or condescending, although in spite of ourselves we would sometimes become interested in an individual patient and exhort him or her to stay sober. In these exhortations we sounded a lot like other "significant others" in our patients' past lives, basing our advice on the false assumption that alcoholics could stay sober if only they wanted to, but in fact expecting very little. Perhaps I was fortunate to have taken a pediatric internship, since it provided less contact

Sheila B. Blume, Medical Director, Alcoholism and Compulsive Gambling Programs, South Oaks Hospital, Amityville, NY.

with patients officially identified as "alcoholic" and therefore less opportunity to absorb negative attitudes from my teachers. In any case, after doing research abroad, I had decided to undertake residency training in psychiatry. It is hard to describe the social milieu of the large state hospital of that era. When I began my training in September, 1962, I became the most junior of a medical staff of about 100, looking after a hospital population of nearly 10,000. The institution itself was much like a small town, with a post office, staff houses, greenhouses, a golf course, a fire house, a police department, and a general hospital, complete with operating rooms and a newborn nursery. All adult patients, regardless of diagnosis or condition, were admitted to one of two admission wards; one male, one female. It was the female admission service to which I was assigned that first day. After a briefing on routine I was handed a list of 25 or 30 names. These were my patients, and I set out to get to know them.

Since I realized it would be impossible to spend a great deal of time with each, I chose the patient I felt was most ill and the one who seemed least ill, and devoted all my available spare time to them in order to learn in greater depth. I knew so little about psychiatry that the patient I chose as "most sick", a young woman with acute schizophrenia, got well rapidly with rest and psychotropic drug treatment, while the patient whom I chose as "least sick", an alcoholic teacher with 6 or 7 children and a difficult marriage—well, she was another story. None of the measures that helped the psychotic patient seemed right for her. There were no psychotropic wonder drugs for alcoholism! Like any good student, when I found myself floundering, I asked for help, and I fully believe that the supervising psychiatrist I consulted set me on my lifelong career in alcoholism with his two word response: "Why bother?"

This man was neither stupid nor lacking in compassion for the mentally ill. He simply reflected the prevalent attitude of the profession of his time. Such patients, in New York in the 1960s, were diagnosed "Without Mental Disorder: Alcoholism, chronic", and were, strictly speaking, supposed to be discharged from the hospital when the diagnosis was made, like any other patient found to be free of mental illness. In fact, they often remained for long periods as voluntary patients, doing unpaid jobs around the hospital, regaining their health and adequate nutrition while they tried to figure out what to do with their lives. The only specific program was a weekly AA meeting on the male ward, for those who wished to attend.

Again, they might be well liked by staff members individually, but were much disliked as a group. My reaction to this attitude was a mixture of shock and disappointment, but it strengthened my resolve to help Mrs. C.

I sought advice where I could find it. I read what was available in the professional literature at the time and had some contact with AA. Because group therapy was recommended by these references, I formed a group of alcoholic women on the admission service by means of trading patients with the other doctors. It was from these women that I acquired my real education.

During my 10 months of service on the female admission ward, the hospital was developing a small experimental alcoholism unit for men on the other side of its multi-acre campus. Shortly after I left the female service, the psychiatrist in charge of this new unit departed for a month and a temporary physician was needed to assist. It is characteristic of the time that not one member of the regular medical staff was willing to accept the assignment. Finally the hospital director recalled that one of the junior trainees actually seemed to enjoy working with alcoholics, so I was asked to do the job. I recall a feeling of pleasurable recognition during my first days there. All of the organizational factors which seemed to be wrong for treating alcoholism on the impersonal, regimented locked admission service were right on this ward. It was open, voluntary and organized to encourage morale and group spirit. I was sure that the hospital really needed a similar program for women.

My first month on D-4 (the unit acquired the name of the small, turn-of-the-century building it inhabited) was a revelation. Although the staff was small (2 doctors, one nurse, one social worker, one counselor, one secretary, and a number of attendants for 60 beds and 500 admissions a year,) the staff worked as a team and worked with AA member volunteers. Treatment was almost always in groups, and rarely did one go by without a good dose of laughter. I asked the nurse to pick out the most "typical alcoholic" on the ward so that I could spend all possible time with him in order to learn. With this man's wife I began to attend open Al-Anon meetings in my home town, incognito. (When I was finally recognized, the members were pleased, but mentioned that I looked a little different from the usual new member because I "didn't have those red eyes!"). Thus I learned about Al-Anon in a very direct way.

When my month was up, I was asked to take charge of the unit, and agreed, but that presented yet another problem. As I was still merely a second year trainee, the other physician refused to work for me, so I had no help. A solution was found in the person of fellow trainee, Dr. John Pitrelli, who had also begun his residency late, but, happily, one day later than I. He was thus technically my junior, and also a friend and one of those rare people whose compassion for patients was not limited to any diagnostic category. John and I, two babes in the woods, undertook to develop the alcoholism program.

It was not easy. We found that the stigma attached to patients rubbed off on those who cared for them. Physicians I otherwise liked and respected would take me aside at parties and advise me to go into some other line, or tell me their method of handling alcoholics ("give them a shovel and a pile of s_____, and you won't see them again!"). We tried to dispel this stigma (and our nickname "the country club") by opening our weekly patient-staff conferences to all hospital personnel, making it part of the regular orientation of new staff and in-service training. I initiated a program psychodrama sessions on the unit, and opened these as well. Later I became director of the hospital's residency training program and saw to it that all psychiatric residents spent time on the unit. We developed a close liaison with the hospital's pastoral counselling training program. In general, we made ourselves available to interested professional groups. At the same time, we went out; to local AA and Al-Anon groups, community groups, professional groups, anyone who would listen. In the late 60s, NBC News made an award-winning television documentary at our unit. These activities both improved our image and kept up our morale.

Alcoholism services in New York State actually owe their beginnings to the 1950 Republican state convention in Saratoga. At a meeting of the platform committee, Colonel Harold Riegelman, a respected statesman, scrawled a sentence on the back of an envelope to the effect that alcoholism should be recognized as a disease and public health problem against which the state would develop a program of control. He based this suggestion on the personal experience of a close friend who had recovered and was active in AA. To his surprise, the plank won unanimous support as the committee members shared similar experiences with friends and family. The Democratic party adopted a similar plank. This initiative found its way into law in 1952 and a number of experimental outpatient programs developed in the '50s under Raymond McCarthy, head of the state's Bureau of Alcoholism within the Department of Mental Hygiene. Colonel Riegelman remained an active and beloved advisor to the State and to the New York City programs until his death, in his 90th year, in 1982.[2]

D-4 was the first experiment in in-patient services in the state hospital system. Thanks to a federal grant from the Hospital Improvement Project, we were able to enrich the D-4 staff and begin the first alcoholism unit for women, called G-5, in 1965. I recall a large all-patient, all-staff discussion with the D-4 patients just before the opening of the new service. Their fantasies were of alcoholic models, actresses and hat-check girls. Actually, in our first year, we treated mostly late middle aged women in fairly advanced stages of the illness, yet a beaten path rapidly developed in the grass between the 2 buildings, over half a mile apart on the campus. Younger women began to arrive in large numbers later on. The two units were joined in 1972.

The success of D-4 and a similar program started shortly afterward at Rochester State Hospital led to the establishment of a statewide network of 17 such state in-patient units, developed in parallel with a larger system of community-based prevention and treatment programs. The firm cooperative relationships initially established with the self-help movement have continued, as has the struggle for public acceptance. After a long political battle in 1978, the Division of Alcoholism broke away from the Department of Mental Hygiene and became a separate agency, its director a member of the Governor's cabinet. The new agency was given the authority to issue alcoholism counselor credentials; fund, certify and manage alcoholism programs, and administer the state's Research Institute on Alcoholism in Buffalo, founded in 1971. I became the director of the Division of Alcoholism in 1979.

Looking back at the 23 years since that first day on the admission ward, I can see a great deal of progress. The 10,000-bed state hospital no longer exists. Well known and successful people now openly identify themselves as having recovered from alcoholism. Public groups have formed to generate support for measures to counteract a variety of alcohol-related problems such as drunken driving. Local Affiliates of the National Council on Alcoholism operate in 200 communities nationwide. AA claims about 25,000 groups and 500,000 members, more and more of them women and young people. Yet the stigma remains. When I meet new people in social situations and tell them what I do, they still giggle nervously and jokingly hide their drinks. When we have talked for a while they will often ask in confidence, "How can you take it? Isn't it depressing?" Depressing? Hardly. I have found a career in alcoholism as stimulating, challenging and rewarding as any to which a physician might aspire. I count myself among the truly fortunate: addicted not to alcohol, but to the study and treatment of alcoholism.

REFERENCES

1. Blume, S. B., *The Alcoholism in Our Patients*, Harvard Medical Alumni Bulletin, December 1980.
2. Blume, S. B. (ed) *The Measure of a Successful Life: An Interview with Colonel Harold Riegelman*, New York State Alcoholism and Alcohol Abuse. Albany, NY, 1982.

Gimme Shelter:
Perspectives on Chronic Inebriates
in Detoxification Centers

Miriam B. Rodin, Ph.D.
Lillian Pickup, RN
Douglas R. Morton, Ph.D.
Carolyn Keatinge, B.A.

Chronic inebriates compose a small but intractable component of the population served by detoxification programs. Both sociological and ethnographic studies of Skid Row populations indicate that the detox system represents a new institution in slum ecology that is readily incorporated into pre-existing patterns of social pathology or adaptation, depending upon the theoretical perspective adopted by the researcher.

Relatively few studies of inebriates have taken an ethnographic perspective. Since Anderson's pioneering study (1923) few new studies were published until the sixties. Skid Row ethnography was revived by Spradley's study of the police inebriates (1970) and by Wiseman (1970) who took a broader view of Skid Row. Ethnography comprised a component of other studies, including those of Bogue (1963), Blumberg et al. (1978), and Bahr and Caplow (1973), though it was distinctly secondary to the social pathology perspective. The first part of this discussion will draw on the ethnographic models of Wiseman and Spradley in order to explain statistical data on inebriates in Chicago. Our findings will lend substantial support to the hypothesis that chronic inebriates incorporate detox into pre-existing patterns of resource exploitation.

Despite the efforts of alcoholism treatment advocates to eliminate the stereotype from public awareness (Room 1976), chronic inebri-

This chapter is based on an earlier paper of the same title presented at the National Council on Alcoholism Annual Forum in Washington, D.C., April 3, 1982. The research was funded in part by a grant from Illinois Department of Mental Health and Development Disabilities Extramural Research Program, Project #839, Demitri B. Shimkin, Ph.D., Department of Anthropology, University of Illinois-Urbana, principal investigator.

ates appear to be objects of policy concern beyond their actual number. That this is so can be attributed to the challenge they present to the disease paradigm of alcoholism underlying current treatment practice. The idea of motivation for treatment has obvious limitations when applied to alcoholism, as a disease of denial. A cornerstone of therapeutic belief in alcoholism treatment is that motivation for recovery is the goal of treatment. Recovery itself involves a long course of sobriety supported by A.A. and other modalities. The chronic inebriate represents the failure of every good intention and therapeutic effort on the part of treatment agencies whose goal is motivation for sobriety. Through repeated failures to maintain sobriety, chronic inebriates have acquired another failure in lives characterized by failure. The attribution of the failure of these men to the treatment system cannot help but frustrate those charged with their rehabilitation. We explore this hypothesis in the second portion of this paper, in which we report the results of a survey of Illinois' detox directors.

To some extent these data may already be anachronistic. Current economic conditions have drastically altered the demography of Skid Row and thus the competitive niche of the chronic inebriate. Large numbers of deinstitutionalized mentally ill and mentally handicapped, homeless elderly and indeed whole families are now competing for the scarce resources of Skid Rows. The inebriates are finding it increasingly difficult. Nonetheless, there is general value in exploring the extent to which the strategies of the homeless put them at odds with the institutions intended to serve—or at least control—them.

Wiseman adopted a widely used analogy of the Skid Row man to a wandering primitive forager. She extended this analogy to an urban transit metaphor of endless cycling through various stations. Fifteen years ago, the principle stations were the jails, the mental hospitals, and the Christian missions. As described by Spradley, the police, courts, and jails were to be avoided, or accommodated by cons and strategems. In Wiseman's account, the mental hospitals and missions offered desirable resources but at the cost of exploitation of work, proximity to the insane, public confessions of sin, and other assaults on the man's mobility and protestations of self-respect. Nonetheless, accommodation to these requirements allowed access to food, shelter, clothing, medical attention, bathing facilities, the company of sympathetic women, male sociability, and sometimes money. Physical safety from the street predators, which was not apparently an important resource at the time of Wiseman's study, has become more important.

In describing the relationship between the alcoholics and the institutions, Wiseman attributed the power of gatekeepers to the institutions, but demonstrated the manipulative capacities of the alcoholics to slide past the gatekeepers to gain access to resources (1970:258). She attributed their successful manipulations to possession of detailed knowledge of system weakness, chinks in the fence of administrative procedures in professional ideologies.

The advent of uniform detoxification acts in many states shifted the institutional structure and resource base available to the alcoholic. In Illinois, and a number of other states, the Acts closed the most desirable station on the loop, the state mental hospital. Within a year of its adoption in Illinois, alcoholism was no longer an admitting diagnosis. The jails have also been closed to the street alcoholic. Thus the power to negotiate diagnostic labels for access to stations formerly within the Skid Row man's power have been lost. Only the alcohol sector is accessible. Furthermore, the involuntary component of the system has been replaced by nearly complete voluntary access through the doors of the short stay detox center.

The Uniform Act defines the point of entry to long stay stations as the detox center. Thus the resources desired by the Skid Row alcoholic: food, shelter, clothing, safety, and so forth are readily available but severely restricted in duration of availability. It is thus not surprising that detox serves the deviance control functions formerly served by the jails, and that the revolving door to jail has been replaced by equal or higher rates of recidivism in detox (Hamilton 1979, Fagan and Mauss 1979, Giesbrecht et al. 1981, Annis and Smart 1978). The Skid Row man thus faces a far simpler array of stations and severely limited powers for self-definition. The effect of the Act with respect to its effectiveness in luring chronic alcoholics into alcohol treatment and ultimately out of the loop has been little evaluated. Table 1 summarizes recent studies of detox utilization patterns.

TRENDS IN CHRONIC INEBRIATE UTILIZATION OF DETOX SERVICES: THE ILLINOIS EXPERIENCE

The studies summarized in Table 1 underline the need to reassess the function of detox centers with regard to chronic inebriates. As well, these studies call into question the appropriateness of defining

Table 1. Summary of Public Inebriate Outcome Studies in the U.S., Canada, and Great Britain, 1955-1981.

Author	Date	Time Span	Facility	Place	Population	n	Findings
Olin	1966	6 month follow-up	Jail	Toronto	chronic drunkards	227	83% ≥ 3 convictions 12% ≥ 36 convictions 77% ≥ 1 hospitalization 40% ≥ 3 hospitalization
Byrne	1967	6 month follow-up	Detox Center	St. Louis	Detox patients	350	25% readmissions
Tyndel	1969	1 year follow-up	Jail	Toronto	chronic drunkards	237	77% ≥ 1 hospitalization 40% ≥ 3 hospitalization 15% ≥ 6 hospitalization
Goldfarb	1970	1 year 1967	Detox Center	Bowery N.Y.	Skid Row alcoholics	1,402	38% readmissions 50% stayed ± 5 days 70% accepted after care referral
Fox et al.	1972	2 years follow-up	Detox Center	Austin	Detox patients	100	43% ≥ 1 readmissions 16% sobriety after 2 years
Gallant et al.	1973	1 year follow-up	Detox Center	New Orleans	compulsory voluntary detox patients	210	50% of patients arrested ≥ 50 times only 17 available on follow-up 6% (sober)
Berns et al.	1974	12 month follow-up	Detox Center	Denver	Detox patients	1,683	56% accepted referral for after care of whom 16% 2 or more readmissions
Garber et al.	1974	1 year	Detox Center	Rochester Minn.	Detox patients	554	33.2% readmission. Average length of stay 44 hrs. 21.9% referred to primary treatment

Table 1. Summary of Public Inebriate Outcome Studies in the U.S., Canada, and Great Britain, 1955-1981.

Author	Date	Time Span	Facility	Place	Population	n	Findings
Annis & Smart	1978	4 month follow-up	3 Detox Centers	Ontario	1st admission Detox patients	522	54% stayed ≥ 5 days, 47% rearrested within 6 months 17% arrested ≥ 4 times 52% at least 1 readmission in 6 months 20% ≥ 3 admission 37% referred to residential treatment of these 66% readmitted to detox 10% confirmed referral to rehab agencies 80% drop out rate overall
Reich & Siegel	1978	1 year	Detox Center	Bowery	Detox patients		60% leave within 10 days
Fagan & Mauss	1979	27-29 month follow-up police records 1970-1976	Detox Center & jails	Seattle	Public inebriates		recidivism 1973 11% recidivism 1975 46% (four fold increase in recidivism)
Hamilton	1979	1 year follow-up	2 Detox Centers & jail	Edinburgh	52 detox patients 48 jail		Detox increase no. of days in hospital 608% ($p < .005$) Increase no. of episodes of drunkness 59% ($p ≤ .05$) Detox did not benefit patients in terms of alcoholism
Giesbrecht et al.	1981	1 year follow-up	Skid Row Services, Police	Toronto	80 Skid Row inebriates 11 administrators 10 policemen		77% Skid Row inebriates been to detox at least once 81% Skid Row inebriates been arrested 42% had increased drinking 48% drank more often 72% believed health was worse

the public inebriate as principally alcoholic or principally homeless. On both medical and ethnographic grounds, the voluntarism of the system may also be questioned. Fox et al. (1972) pointed out that a short stay results in discharging the inebriate during the post-withdrawal period of heightened arousal, during which time he is most likely to seek relief in drinking again. These authors suggested mandatory stays of seven to ten days in order to capitalize on post-withdrawal psychological dependency needs. Wiseman's ethnography also argues for increased lengths of stay in order to control exploitative demands on care providers.

The majority of studies cited have reported on one year or less of follow-up experience. Thus the extent to which Skid Row inebriates have incorporated the detox centers into pre-existing patterns of adaptation and exploitation has not been fully assessed. In Illinois, a long sequence of admissions data are available through the Department of Mental Health and Developmental Disabilities Division of Alcoholism. A decriminalization statute was implemented in July, 1976. Shortly thereafter, and in part responsive to Federal concerns expressed in the NIAAA conference report of 1981, data are separately prepared on clients meeting an a priori definition of recidivism. Those meeting the definition include individuals admitted ten or more times in a single year to one program. Table 2 summarizes five and one-half years' admissions experience in Illinois, comparing recidivists to all admissions among twenty-four reporting agencies. Overall these data are consistent both with NIAAA national pilot data (1981a), and with the single city or single agency studies reviewed earlier. As shown, both total number of clients served and the proportion of clients meeting the Illinois definition of recidivism peaked in 1979, when recidivists accounted for 8.3% of clients and slightly over a quarter of all admissions. The proportions of recidivists among all clients declined slowly thereafter, as did the relative proportion of admissions that they represented. These data suggest several possible and not mutually exclusive explanations.

Examination of the demographic characteristics over time shows that in the first few years, the Skid Row-like character of recidivists increased. When compared to all clients they were more likely chronically unemployed, transient, undomiciled and brought in by the police. Thereafter, the proportions brought in by the police declined among recidivists, but remain stable among all clients. The proportion unemployed and undomiciled after 1979 remained higher among recidivists than among all clients, but declined somewhat as well. Further, the proportion of all clients referred to hospitals, alcohol treatment, or residential care remain constant throughout, but the proportion of recidivist admissions resulting in referral rose through 1980 and declined thereafter. These data support Nimmer's (1971) hypothesis of decreasing police cooperation over time. The reduction in police transportations thus reduced the number of incapacitated admissions but did not likely affect the behavior of those Wiseman has characterized as purposeful users of service. The decline in repeater referrals per admission may indicate a shift in detox staff policies or in client behavior. That is, detox centers may have cut off access to rehabilitation stations. Thus, although the proportions of admissions of recidivist clients that resulted in referral declined, the sheer numbers of referrals that they could obtain need not have declined. That is, with persistent and repeated entry into the detox system, chronic inebriates can overcome administrative resistance and force their way into desirable long stay stations. Alternatively, reduction of numbers of recidivists may represent the creaming of motivated clients in earlier years leaving a hard core

Table 2: Statistical Summary of Social Detoxication Programs, Client Characteristics and Utilization Among All Clients and Repeaters in Illinois July 1, 1976 to June 31, 1982.

	FY 77		FY 78		FY 79	
	All	Rptrs	All	Rptrs	All	Rptrs
No. of Clients	12,124	468	15,300	662	15,290	502
No. of Admissions	32,448	10,168	43,583	15,651	39,705	13,051
Percent Male	91.9	98.5	92.4	98.8	91.2	98.8
Percent White	69.8	64.7	64.3	63.1	63.6	63.3
Percent Undomiciled and Transient	26.6	57.9	34.8	66.2	32.0	72.7
Percent Unemployed	23.8	34.3	30.3	52.9	41.9	74.3
Percent police transport	53.3	73.4	52.3	66.6	52.4	72.3
Percent given referral	21.4	8.3	19.5	8.4	20.3	10.1

Source: State of Illinois Department of Mental Health and Developmental Disabilities. Division of Alcoholism. Statistical Summary of Social Setting Detoxication Programs. July 1, 1977 through December 31, 1981.

Table 2: Statistical Summary of Social Detoxication Programs, Client Characteris-
          tics and Utilization Among All Clients and Repeaters in Illinois
          July 1, 1976 to June 31, 1982

	FY 80		FY 81		FY 82 (1st 6 months)	
	All	Rptrs	All	Rptrs	All	Rptrs
No. of Clients	15,158	420	14,904	292	8,229	127
No. of Admissions	34,383	8,992	30,387	5,640	15,794	2,355
Percent Male	90.5	97.9	90.5	97.9	90.7	97.6
Percent White	62.7	64.8	62.5	67.1	62.1	58.3
Percent Undomiciled and Transient	31.2	69.1	24.6	51.0	24.1	57.5
Percent Unemployed	37.9	53.8	35.0	56.2	34.6	66.1
Percent police transport	44.4	57.6	33.5	39.4	32.2	37.2
Percent given referral	21.6	13.0	22.0	8.3	20.3	6.9

Source: State of Illinois Department of Mental Health and Developmental Disabili-
         ties. Division of Alcoholism.
         Statistical Summary of Social Setting Detoxication Programs. July 1, 1977
         through December 31, 1981.

residual group. Finally, the changes may simply reflect overall
decreases in the chronic pool through dispersal of Skid Row populations and differential mortality. In the following discussion these
possibilities will be addressed, although conclusions are necessarily
somewhat speculative.

THE EFFECT OF REFERRAL TO TREATMENT:
A TEST OF THE ADAPTATION
WITHOUT REHABILITATION HYPOTHESIS

To determine whether the decrease in statewide referrals reflected successful rehabilitation of clients or an accommodation between administrative resistance to referral and chronic inebriates'
strategy of persistence, one detox center was selected for further
study. Nearly all Illinois detox admissions originated in urban areas
throughout the State, with two-thirds of these reported from four

Chicago centers. The ATA Detox Center in Uptown, a Chicago Skid Row area, is operated by Lutheran Social Services Alcohol and Drug Dependency Programs by contract to the state. Utilization and client characteristics for the years July 1, 1978 through June 30, 1979 are comparable to state-wide data. Comparison of the two years demonstrated shifts in the directions observed state-wide. One thousand nine hundred forty-one clients accounted for 5152 admissions to ATA in Financial Year (FY) 1980. Of these, 86 were admitted ten or more times in that year, but 239 (2.3%) had had ten or more admissions since July 1, 1976 as determined by record review. Of all FY 1980 admissions, 783 (15.2%) resulted in 114 placements in alcohol treatment programs, four referrals to state mental hospitals, 663 referrals to general medical hospitals, and two placements in ATA in-house residential programs. The remainder of clients were discharged home (14.6%), to AA (1.5%), or to "other" (68.4%). "Other" included a mixed group of shelters, missions, VA hospitals and self-discharged against staff advice. Thus extrapolating back to state-wide data, the apparent increase in non-referral among recidivists apparently understated the likelihood that a detox admission would result in procurement of referrals to sources of food and shelter.

For the referral study, ATA records of all admissions remaining at least 24 hours in the holding area in calendar year 1979 were pulled. From these, all admissions resulting in a firm referral were selected and unduplicated, resulting in a total of 374 clients having obtained at least one firm referral during the year. A firm referral was defined as both client acceptance of referral and receiving agency acceptance of the client as indicated by reservation of bed for an agreed upon date. For time dependent analyses, the index was set at the date of the first 1979 admission resulting in a firm referral. A control group was then selected from the admitting log after removal of the 374 referred clients. Every fourth referred client was matched from the admitting log to the next client admitted on the index date who did not obtain a firm referral during 1979. One hundred and eighty-five control client records were abstracted. We then had up to 2-1/2 years previous admission and referral history and up to 1-1/2 years of follow-up. Demographic, drinking history, and social function measures on a total of 559 detox clients were also obtained. In logistic regression analyses, twenty clients were excluded because the number of admissions was so extreme (over one hundred in one case) that statistical tests dependent upon mean values were rendered meaningless. In the logistic analysis a further 72 records were excluded due to incomplete data on demographic variables. The groups are compared in Table 3. Referred clients had an average of 4.9 as compared with 2.9 admissions to detox, or an average of two more admissions than did the control clients admitted on the same day. This supports the hypothesis that by increasing his number of admissions, a repeater increases his likelihood of obtaining referral. Being unmarried and having veteran's benefits also correlated with obtaining referral. Merging the referred and control groups, we partitioned the total sample into categories of one, two to ten and eleven or more admissions. In that order, the mean age of the groups increased, as did the

Table 3: Detox Center Utilization and Demographic Characteristics of ATA
          Referred and Non-Referred Groups, 1979.

Utilization	Referred (N=374)	Not Referred (N=185)	All (N=559)
Mean no. of admissions prior to index	4.0	3.8	3.9
Mean no. of admissions subsequent to index*	4.9	2.9	4.2
Mean total admissions 1976-1980	9.9	7.8	9.2
Mean no. of total referrals 1976-80*	1.8	0.4	1.4
Average length of stay per admission (days)	2.9	2.7	2.8

Demographic Characteristics			
Mean age (years)	41.3	42.4	41.6
Mean years of schooling	10.9	10.8	10.9
Percent employed at least part-time	12.2	18.1	14.1
Percent male*	95.7	87.5	93.0
Percent white*	63.8	68.9	65.5
Percent married*	5.8	14.5	8.5
Percent veteran*	52.9	30.5	45.9
Mean years of heavy drinking reported	12.7	14.4	13.1

* Differences significant at p < .05 or better as computed by X^2 or F-test as appropriate.

Source: State of Illinois Department of Mental Health and Developmental
         Disabilities. Division of Alcoholism. Statistical Summary of
         Social Setting Detoxication Programs. July 1, 1977 through
         December 31, 1981.

proportion of white, unmarried, unemployed and undomiciled males. The proportions increased as well of those having prior inpatient alcoholism treatment, and those receiving further referrals subsequent to the index admission.

We next attempted to go beyond published studies of recidivism among detox clients by directly assessing the impact of further treatment by referral. Detox and referral history, demographic characteristics, and additional variables including drinking history and number of medical and social function problems on index intake (fifteen variables in all) were entered into a multiple logistic regression. The outcome measure selected was readmission to detox. As shown in Table 4, five variables contributed significantly to readmission. The algorithm was then run forward to test the predictive power of the combined variables shown in Table 4. Our model correctly identified recidivists in 84.6% of cases and correctly identified non-recidivists in slightly more than half of all cases (54.6%). In all the model correctly classified recidivists and non-recidivists 73.7% of the time. The combination of high prior utilization of detoxification services and a demographic profile including being unmarried, unemployed, undomiciled and displaying poor social function accurately predicted recidivism. It is further significant, in light of the above reporting of an association between obtaining a referral and subsequently increased numbers of detox admissions, that the fact of referral was not a significant contributor to the regression algorithm.

Thus, much as the survival patterns described by Wiseman, the present strategy appears to be one of persistence. Whether this is motivated by rational utility as implied by the interactionist framework adopted by Wiseman, or by the learned expectation of failure proposed much earlier by Rubington (1958) and amplified by the clinical considerations offered by Fox et al. (1972) cannot be answered by these data. Nonetheless it is important to note the conspicuous absence of clinical factors such as length of heavy drinking, medical condition or prior alcoholism among the significant predictors of recidivism. We now turn to an assessment of the treatment system response to the strategy of persistence.

ILLINOIS DETOX DIRECTORS SURVEY, 1982

In 1982, a variety of organizational factors led to a statewide survey of detox directors to which we added open-ended questions designed to elicit the extent to which the chronic client affected staff

Table 4:   Multiple Logistic Analysis of Factors Predicting Readmission
           to ATA Detox (N=467)

Variable	Beta	x^2	p	D
Intercept	-.27	2.41	.12	-
No. of admissions prior to index	.21	25.95	.0001	.053
Undomiciled	.79	13.14	.0003	.028
Currently Married	-.92	4.64	.0311	.010
Currently employed	-.63	4.70	.0302	.010
Social Problem Score	.65	10.40	.0013	.022
Total Model		93.73 (5 df)	.0001	.169

morale. There were 24 detox centers in Illinois at that time, four in Chicago, three in the Chicago suburbs and the rest downstate. We first elicited staff definitions of recidivism.

The state definition of a recidivist was more than ten admissions per year to one facility. Detox directors were asked for their definitions. Three directors defended the disease paradigm, stating they did not see any such clients or that any such definition was irrelevant to treatment; although two subsequently described a "Skid Row" profile in response to other questions. Directors varied considerably in their perceptions. Several downstate directors considered any return to a center as recidivism. Two Chicago directors felt a recidivist had to have at least 30 admissions in a year to qualify for the title.

We probed the problem a second way by asking directors to what extent they admitted clients not for treatment but for shelter. Five directors said they never did. Nineteen stated that anywhere from "a few" to "most" of their admissions were to provide temporary shelter not treatment to inebriates.

As stated earlier, fewer than 10% of detox clients fit the state definition of recidivism in any year. We asked directors to estimate the number of homeless alcoholics they knew of in their service areas, regardless of whether they were admitted to treatment. Five directors in two rural regions could not answer; two directors reported that there were none. In both of the latter cases, independent observation argued for the presence of street alcoholics in the communities but their exclusion from the center. The remaining directors estimated a total of 320 chronic inebriates, about evenly split between Chicago and the rest of the state. This approximates closely the number obtained from 1981-1982 admissions data reported in Table 2, although different individuals may have been counted in each case.

That the repeaters or recidivists had endangered a profound threat to the treatment paradigm emerged from another question in which directors were asked to name additional services they felt were needed. One director desired the power to refuse admission. Eighteen more specifically named no-treatment alternatives. Their responses fell evenly into two groups, half suggesting non-treatment care in voluntary shelters and wet hotels. In other words half the directors favored a return to a version of the urban mission. Of those preferring involuntary commitment, five specifically named involuntary three-day hold or commitment. Four more suggested extended stay, custodial "farms". These responses indicate a return to the mental hospital model of care.

The detox director survey indicates the presence of a challenge to the treatment paradigm engendered by a small number of chronic street alcoholics. It seems as though the alcoholics' definition of the situation has forced a rethinking of the approach to treatment, if only because of the sheer magnitude of their demands upon the system for food and shelter, but evidently not sobriety.

The Illinois Detox Center Directors survey indicates a rather profound shift away from a unitary paradigm of treatment. At the outset, the dominant disease model offered the promise of rehabilitation through detoxification and referral. Both the quantitative data and the detox directors' perspectives demonstrate failure of the model with respect to a small group of chronics. Yet the conflict engendered by their presence seems to go further. The individual orientation toward treatment is based on psychological or biological theories of etiology and issues of individual patient motivation for sobriety. Sociological theorists have, on the other hand, supported the view that drinking and revolving door use of detox is consistent with social structural and socialization etiologies and with community based interventions. The effect on the morale of detox center line-staff, often recovering alcoholics themselves with minimal training, cannot help but be demoralizing. The cost in staff demoralization, turnover, and frustration has been little addressed in the published literature.

In addition to our own study however, this effect is being recognized. Stall (1982) for example has stated that "the definition of recidivism by the staff as a "major treatment problem" could not have been better chosen to make apparent the differences between the disease and social models of alcoholism" (1982:15). In research conducted in the Lexington, Kentucky Center he found that recovering counselors trained in disease model approaches of confrontation and counseling sessions focused on drinking resulted in shorter stays by recidivists, counteracting the accepted view of clinical researchers that longer stay in detox exerts beneficial effects. Weibel-Orlando reports similar findings in a study of a center for American Indians in Los Angeles, where the "ideal model" of stages of recovery is subverted by chronic inebriate clients who do not recognize the ritual progressions, but utilize the treatment system as a method for sustaining long ingrained patterns such as those we have discussed using Wiseman's framework (1982:14). The largely Indian staff, thus experienced as high as 90% failure rates among their charges, and thus faced the frustration of continually initiating "flawed rites of passage." Both authors recommend reconsideration of the appropriateness of alcoholism rehabilitation based upon the disease model among chronic inebriates.

By many accounts then, it appears that the detox system is faced with a choice of accepting the chronic inebriates' definition of it as a station on the loop or to choose to diversify therapeutic approaches. To the extent that successful efforts have been reported they are based on the sociocultural model of Skid Row drinking as a way of life. Rather than redefining detox as a gateway to missions and farms as did the Illinois directors, several alternative models have been proposed. In the Vera Institute project on the Bowery, sobriety was initially secondary to building dependence upon staff in supported living over a year or more. By entering men into stable residential groups and gradually increasing demands for self-support through work and house self-government, men were slowly resocialized. Relocation away from Skid Row, again in supported living groups, was attempted in Philadelphia. Siegal (1978) reported on treating existing living groups in SRO hotels as social clients. In this case, individual therapy and sobriety were distinctly secondary to enhancing the aggregate ability to achieve more satisfactory life adjustments.

The extent to which such community-based social model approaches have been adopted is as yet rather limited, and little is known about their long-term effectiveness in reintegrating chronic inebriates more acceptable life styles. Their existence however, does suggest a shift in paradigms from the focus on individual alcoholism to recognition of recidivism as a social adaptation that may be vulnerable to social intervention. A great deal of further social and ethnographic research is needed to establish the validity of this "diagnosis" and the reliability of indicators in selecting cases. However, if the detoxification system is to withstand both internal doubt and external attack fostered by the continued presence of the chronic inebriate, a resolution must be sought.

REFERENCES

Anderson, Nels *The Hobo: The Sociology of the Homeless Man* (Chicago: University of Chicago Press, 1923).

Annis, Helen M. and Reginald Smart "Arrests, Readmissions and Treatment Following Release From Detoxification Centers" *Journal of Studies on Alcohol* 39 (1978): 1276-1283.

Bahr, Howard M. and Theodore Caplow *Old Men Drunk and Sober* (New York: New York University Press, 1973).

Berns, Barry R. and Stephen L. Dilts "Denver's Detoxification Unit" *Rocky Mountain Medical Journal* April (1974): 220-222.

Blumberg, Leonard, Thomas E. Shipley and Stephen F. Barsky *Liquor and Poverty: Skid Row as a Human Condition* (New Brunswick, N.J.: Publications Division, Rutgers Center of Alcohol Studies, 1978).

Bogue, Donald J. *Skid Row in American Cities* (Chicago: Community and Family Study Center, University of Chicago, 1963).

Byrne, Robert J. "Detoxification . . . An Emergency Apostolate" *Hospital Progress* 48 (1967): 86-89.

Fagan, Ronald W. and Armand L. Mauss "Padding the Revolving Door: An Initial Assessment of the Uniform Alcoholism and Intoxication Treatment Act in Practice," *Social Problems* 26 (1979): 230-246.

Fox, Richard P., Marie B. Graham and Michael J. Gill "A Therapeutic Revolving Door" *Archives of General Psychiatry* 26 (1972): 179-182.

Gallant, Donald M. et al. "The Revolving-Door Alcoholic" *Archives of General Psychiatry* 28 (1973): 633-635.

Garber, J. J., E. V. Dolander and J. D. Dexter "Alcoholic Detoxification: A One Year Experience" *Minnesota Medicine* (February, 1974): 143-145.

Giesbrecht, Norman A., P. James Giffen, Sylvia Lambert and Gus Oki "Changes in the Social Control of Skid Row Inebriates in Toronto: Assessments by Skid Row Informants" *Canadian Journal of Public Health* 72 (1981): 101-104.

Goldfarb, Charles "Patients Nobody Wants—Skid Row Alcoholics" *Diseases of the Nervous System* 31 (1970): 274-281.

Hamilton, John R. "Evaluation of a Detoxification Service for Habitual Drunken Offenders" *British Journal of Psychiatry* 135 (1979): 28-34.

National Institute of Alcohol Abuse and Alcoholism *An Evaluation Report of N.I.A.A.A.: Public Inebriate Programs (P.I.P.) for Fiscal Year 1980* (Evaluation Brief #22, Program Analysis and Evaluation Branch, 1981).

National Institute of Alcohol Abuse and Alcoholism *An Evaluation Report of N.I.A.A.A.: Public Inebriate Issues* (Conference Report, 1981).

Nimmer, Raymond T. *Two Million Unnecessary Arrests: Removing a Social Service Concern from the Criminal Justice System* (Chicago: American Bar Foundation, 1971).

Olin, Jack A. " 'Skid Row' Syndrome: A Medical Profile of the Chronic Drunkenness Offender" *Canadian Medical Association Journal* 95 (1966): 205-214.

Reich, Robert and Lloyd Siegal "The Emergence of the Bowery as a Psychiatric Dumping Ground" *Psychiatric Quarterly* 50 (1978): 191-201.

Room, Robin "Comment" *Journal of Studies on Alcohol* 37 (1976): 113-144.

Rubington, Earl "The Chronic Drunkenness Offender" *Annals of the American Academy of Political and Social Science* 315 (1958): 65-72.

Siegal, Harvey A. *Outpost of the Forgotten: Socially Terminal People in Slum Hotels and Single Room Occupancy Tenements* (New Brunswick, N.J.: Transaction Books, 1978).

Spradley, James P. *You Owe Yourself a Drunk: An Ethnography of Urban Nomads* (Boston: Little Brown and Company., 1978).

Stall, Ronald D. "Disadvantages of Eclecticism in the Treatment of Alcoholism: The 'Problem' of Recidivism" Paper presented at the Society for Applied Anthropology, Lexington, Ky, 1982.

State of Illinois Department of Mental Health and Developmental Disabilities, Division of Alcoholism "Statistical Summary of Social Setting Detoxification Programs, July 1, 1977 through December 31, 1981."

Tyndel, Milo "Psychiatric Study of the Chronic Drunkenness Offender" *Canadian Psychiatric Association Journal* 14 (1969): 275-285.

Weibel-Orlando, Joan C. "Alcoholism Treatment Programs as Flawed Rites of Passage" Paper presented at the Society for Applied Anthropology, Lexington, Ky, 1982.

Wiseman, Jacqueline P. *Stations of the Lost: The Treatment of Skid Row Alcoholics* (Chicago: University of Chicago Press, 1970).

Staff Culture
and Public Detoxes

Earl Rubington

Public detoxes have to accept most of the clients who come to their doors for service. Since recent state laws specify that alcoholics are sick people, not criminals, detox clients are free to decide if they need detoxification, to leave any time they wish, and to return frequently for multiple detoxifications (Fagan and Mauss, 1978). Having been given little control over readmission or retention of clients by law, detox goals of helping, sustaining, and changing their clients have been placed in jeopardy. How public detoxes regulate readmission, retention, and influence of clients is the subject of this paper.

Detox studies have arrived at some fairly general conclusions (Annis and Smart, 1978; Fagan and Mauss, 1978; Daggett and Rolde, 1977; Den Hartog, 1982; Regier, 1979; Rodin and others, 1985; Udell and Hornstra, 1975; and Westermeyer and Lang, 1975). Detox clients have not responded in ways alcoholism planners had expected. Most stay only a very short time, frequently leave before treatment has been completed, relapse shortly after discharge, and return again and again for detoxification. Very few continue treatment begun in detox. And those few, similarly, maintain minimal contact with treatment agencies to which they have been referred and also relapse at a very high rate.

Most of these studies explain detox outcomes by the social characteristics of their typical clients, the chronic public inebriates. Few of them look at problems clients present, staff ways of solving these problems, and if these ways shape detox outcomes.

Do public detoxes try to get their clients to stay in the detoxes longer? What do they try to do about the problem of readmissions?

Earl Rubington, Department of Sociology and Anthropology, Northeastern University, Boston, Massachusetts.

This research was supported by Grant AA 02900 from the National Institute of Alcohol Abuse and Alcoholism.

What success, if any, have they had in retaining clients while decreasing readmissions? How do they influence their clients to make changes in their lives? And in what ways are these influences related to post-detox referrals?

This exploratory study suggests that the kinds of interactions that take place in public detoxes may answer some of these questions. Detox staff interact with fellow-staff, the detox director, and the array of clients who come in and out. Since these interactions present fairly recurrent problems, staff devise ways of dealing with problem clients, fellow-staff members, and detox directors make for them. Shared ways of defining, interpreting, and responding to recurrent problems make up staff culture. Where previous studies explain results by characteristics of clients, this exploration argues that staff ways need to be included when explaining both detox processes and outcomes.

This paper advances the cultural argument to supplement rather than replace the characteristics-of-detox-clients explanation. First it presents ethnographic evidence on how six public detoxes seek to decrease readmissions and to increase retention. Then it looks at the relationship between these controls on clients and readmission and retention rates. Next it describes how these public detoxes counsel clients. And then it explores the relationship between these different ways of influencing clients and post-detox referrals. It concludes with a typology of detox cultures and then suggests some changes which may simplify detox process, raise staff morale, and, possibly improve outcomes.

SETTING

Since all six public detoxes do medical detoxification, a description of this model will help in understanding similarities and differences in the six detoxes.

There are eight steps in this model: referral, screening, intake, withdrawal, care, counseling, convalescence, and discharge. *Referral:* Clients or other sources call detox and ask if a bed is available. A nurse, an aide, or a clerk takes the call, and, if a bed is available, asks a few questions. If they decide to accept the candidate, they tell the caller they will hold the bed for two hours. *Screening:* On arrival, a nurse asks the candidate a few questions about the present drinking episode, drinking and drug history, illnesses and injuries, and then decides whether to admit the client. If she thinks the person "needs detoxification," she admits. *Intake:* Once admitted, an aide takes over, fills out several forms, stores clothing and valuables, showers the client, and then escorts him to the examining room. *Withdrawal:* The nurse gives the client a complete physical examination, takes a detailed medical history which includes questions on use of alcohol and other drugs, and then starts the treatment of alcohol withdrawal, usually with a prescribed dosage of Librium. The aide then escorts the client to an assigned bed. *Care:* Aides take vital signs (blood pressure, pulse, respiration, and temperature) every four hours. As the client "comes down," the nurse administers decreasing doses of Librium (according to a reduction cure formula prescribed by the medical director) and treats minor medical problems. On the second day in detox a counselor gathers a history of drinking and previous treatments for alcoholism. This becomes the basis in subsequent discussions with the client for working out a post-detox alcoholism treatment plan such as referral to a halfway house, in-patient residential facility, out-patient alcoholism clinic, Alcoholics Anonymous, mental health clinic, etc. *Convalescence:* Once clients can walk, they attend morning, afternoon, and evening meetings such as "rap sessions," films, slide shows, resource meetings and AA meetings. *Discharge:* Upon completion of treatment which should last at least five days, clients get clothing and valuables back, dress, sign necessary forms and leave detox. If taking placement, a detox vehicle transports them to the facility.

THE SIX PUBLIC DETOXES

Summary descriptions of the six public detoxes follow below and include ecology, physical plant, clientele, and staff.

North*

Established by a grant from LEAA in 1971, North Detox is located in the West End, a neighborhood known for its many unattached males and numerous arrests for drunkenness. The largest of Metro City's detoxes, North has 56 beds and occupies seven floors of one wing of a large residential hotel. A school, a park, some light industry, and private dwelling places surround it. It is only a block

---

*Names of persons or places are fictitious.

away from Metro City Hospital where it sends any clients who need immediate medical attention and from whose alcoholism clinic it receives (as do all the other detoxes) numerous clients for detoxification. North Detox's street rescue team patrols West End streets in a van looking for voluntary candidates for detoxification. In the beginning most of its clients came in by way of street rescue, police drop-off, emergency services, or other alcoholism treatment programs. But at the time of this study, most clients were self-referred. Most of them came in through the Metro City Alcoholism Clinic. North's clients, predominantly older, unattached and indigent chronic public inebriates came mainly from the West End. In all, some fifty full-time and part-time staff worked at North Detox and their average age was 29. A thirty-year-old nonalcoholic woman directed operations. The ratio of nonalcoholics to recovering alcoholics on its staff was 3:2.

South

Opened in 1973, South Detox is located in a commercial, nonresidential area. It rents a first-floor wing of a building owned and operated by American Rescue Missionaries, a religious organization. ARM operates its own shelter and alcoholism treatment facilities in the main building. South, unlike the other detoxes in these respects, concentrates all of its space on one small ground floor, detoxifies men only, and has no kitchen or dining room. Ambulatory clients take their meals upstairs in the ARM cafeteria. Like all the other detoxes in this study (except for North), it has 20 beds. Its four major sources of referral are self, Metro City Alcoholism Clinic (a mile and a half away), in-patient alcoholism programs, and residential alcoholism programs, in that order. Chronic public inebriates who predominate among its clients come in from all sections of the city including the West End. Its chronic inebriate population is somewhat older than North's. Its staff averages 29 years, the ratio of alcoholics to nonalcoholics is 4:2. At the time of this study, a 35-year-old nonalcoholic male directed its staff of 20.

West

Opened in September, 1973, West occupies two floors of a former convent in a lower-middle-class residential neighborhood. The first floor consists of administrative offices, offices for admission clerk, director, administrative assistant, alcoholism counselors, pantry, and dining facilities. On the second floor, there is a four-bed intensive care unit, eight two-bed rooms, dayroom, nurses' station, staff meeting room, lavatory and utility room. West's clients are predominantly walk-ins. Otherwise, they come from other alcoholism programs or the Metro City Alcoholism Clinic (some 3-1/4 miles away). Its clients are mainly unattached, blue-collar alcoholics in the 35-50 age range, older chronic public inebriates between 51 and 65, and a few older unattached white-collar alcoholics. At the time of the study some 25 people worked in West Detox and their average age was 35. The ratio of nonalcoholics to alcoholics was 2:2. West's middle-aged director was a recovering alcoholic who had regained his sobriety in O'Brien House (not far from West) and who had worked as an alcoholism counselor in East Detox for two years before assuming the directorship of West Detox.

East

East Detox, which opened February, 1974, also occupies a remodeled convent in a working-class neighborhood. Cooking and cleaning facilities are in the basement. Waiting room, admitting office, offices for director, counselors, and nursing supervisor, dayroom, dining room and pantry are all on the second floor. Examining room, nurses' station, staff meeting room, 10-bed intensive care unit, and four bedrooms for ambulatory clients are all on the second floor. East Detox clients come mainly as self-referrals from the Metro City Alcoholism Clinic (four miles away), and from other alcoholism programs. They are generally chronic public inebriates from the surrounding neighborhood or from the West End, generally in the 35-50 age range, unattached, blue-collar alcoholics in their 40s, and a smaller cadre of white-collar alcoholics generally of the same age. Some 35 people work in East Detox and their average age is 32. There are two recovering alcoholics on the staff for every three nonalcoholics. Its 45-year-old director was a recovering alcoholic who had regained his sobriety in Sober House, a halfway house some ten blocks away. After serving as head alcoholism counselor at East, he was promoted to director when its director resigned in 1976.

Northeast

Opened in August, 1974, Northeast Detox operates in what used to be a two-story nursing home in a predominantly black community. Examining room, 8-bed intensive care unit, nursing and counselors' offices, utility rooms, kitchen, and dayroom are all on the first floor. Six two-bed rooms are on the second floor for ambulatory patients. A wall separates patients from four offices: two for secretaries, one each for the director, and his administrative assistant. Northeast clients are mainly self-referrals, from minority alcoholism programs as well as other alcoholism programs. All candidates for detoxification must first obtain medical clearance at the Metro City Alcoholism Clinic (some two miles away) before they can gain admission. Fifty percent of its clients are black. Its black clients are younger, mostly in the 35-50 age category, and predominantly unattached blue-collar alcoholics. Its white clients, generally older chronic public inebriates, come from other sections of the city. At the time of the study, 20 people worked at Northeast Detox. One was a white staff nurse, the rest were all blacks. The ratio of nonalcoholics to alcoholics was six to two. Its director was a middle-aged recovered alcoholic who had regained his sobriety in a minority halfway house called Struggle some ten blocks away.

Southwest

Opened in June, 1975, Southwest Detox occupies a separate two-story building on the grounds of a chronic disease hospital. At one end of the first floor corridor there is a large nurse's station, a small examining office and two 10-bed wards on either side of the nurses' station. At the other end of the corridor is the dayroom and adjoining kitchen. One enters the first floor in the center of this corridor. There is an admitting office just to the right of the entrance. Record room, meeting rooms, administrative and counselors' offices are all on the second floor. Southwest clients come in mainly as self-referrals or from the Metro City Alcoholism Clinic (5-1/2 miles away). The next largest source of referrals in order are alcoholism programs (emergency services, in-patient, or out-patient). Older blue-collar alcoholics, generally unattached, come from the surrounding neighborhood. These clients, mostly in their middle fifties, make up about 40% of the clientele. Older, attached, white-collar alcoholics, in their late 50s or early 60s comprise the remaining twenty percent. The twenty people who work at Southwest average 36 years of age and half of them are recovering alcoholics. Its director, at the time of this study, was a middle-aged nonalcoholic.

METHOD

Data for this study come from two months' fieldwork in each of the detoxes. Fieldwork (observation, interviewing, and examination of detox records) focused primarily on intake, counseling, and discharge. Observation of staff processing clients included intake interviews, medical screenings, and discharge procedures. Observation of staff and others preparing clients for post-detox treatment roles included attendance at "rap sessions" and resource meetings (as when visiting halfway house personnel described what their facilities had to offer to clients leaving detox) and, of course, AA meetings. Additional observation of staff included case conferences (in which staff discussed clients' progress and made plans for medicating, monitoring, counseling, formulating post-detox plans, referring, and discharging clients). Interviews, both formal and informal, centered on the counseling process, procedure and records, and varieties of clients and their problems. Detox records included admission log, nurses' log, nurses' notes, counselors' notes, and client files.

Case records provided the data for analysis of length of stay, percentage of readmissions, and kinds of discharge. Each detox admission log contains some of the following facts on every admission: name, date admitted, source of referral, number of previous admissions, day discharged, and kind of discharge. Clients leave detox in three ways (TP, OP, and AMA), all of which coincide with staff rank-ordering of preferred discharges. If clients accept a post-detox referral to another alcoholism treatment facility (in-patient, out-patient, or residential), this was called "took placement" or TP. If clients stayed the minimum 5 days and left without post-detox referrals, this was called "own plan" or OP. If clients left before their treatment was considered completed, this was called "against medical advice" or AMA. The normative ranking of these three kinds of discharges can be seen in the following way: clients who left "took placement" had gotten medical help and accepted detox influences to continue the process of self-change. Clients who left "own plan" received full medical treatment but may or may not have responded to the counseling staff's pressure to continue changes begun in the detox. And, finally, clients who left "against medical advice" neither completed the medical treatment nor accepted any advice on what to do about their drinking problem after discharge.

For comparative purposes, information was collected on all clients who had come into and left any of the six detoxes one or more times during the same two months' study period. Length of stay, percentages of readmissions, and kinds of discharges form the basis of the analysis of treatment outcomes which follows.

THE PROBLEM OF RETENTION AND READMISSION

Because they are public facilities, public detoxes have very little to say about the clients who seek their services. When the alcoholism movement defined alcoholics as sick people rather than as criminals, it gave clients more power to decide if and when they wish treatment, how long they will stay in treatment, and how often they will return for treatment. This shift in the balance of power gave all public detoxes their problems of retention and readmission.

This paper argues that staff culture offers solutions to these two important problems. Accordingly, it first describes alternate ways of solving these problems. Then it examines how these ways of coping affect retention and readmission.

Brief descriptions of how each detox tried to deal with these recurrent problems follow. The summaries center on what staff said about these issues during the fieldwork period; whether their policies stressed retention, readmission, both, or neither; whether detox staff disagreed about these policies and, if so, how they resolved the conflicts (if at all); and, lastly, how uniformly staff applied these decision rules on retention and readmission.

North Detox

North Detox's rescue team caused persistent staff conflict over admissions. Frequently, the rescue team brought in potential clients whom medical personnel refused to admit. The medical screening person often rejected candidates recently discharged from North Detox who had not been drinking long enough to risk either acute intoxication or severe withdrawal symptoms. Additionally, medical personnel sometimes felt that rescue brought in former drinking acquaintances who needed shelter for the night more than detoxification.

Rescue saw their task in criminal justice terms, while medical staff more often saw their role as a public health one (Shire and Smith, 1976). Rescue believed they were supposed to remove intoxicated persons who were at risk of arrest by police, get them detoxified, and then offer them "a shot at rehabilitation." Medical staff preferred to service candidates who had a better prognosis of recovery from alcoholism or who, at the least, were experiencing relatively severe withdrawal distress. North Detox, a new facility within the changing system of alcoholism treatment services, did not always give either rescue or medical staff equal opportunity to act on their preferences. Even before decriminalization of public drunkenness in the state, admissions and discharges were wholly voluntary. Alcoholics, now sick rather than criminal, were free to come into and leave treatment as they chose despite what detox staff might feel.

Two recovered alcoholic staff members (one, the assistant director, the other, the head counselor) both said publicly and with considerable pride that North Detox, unlike all the other public detoxes in the state, did not have a "black list." The pride they felt contrasted sharply with a medical staff who felt the situation was tantamount to "open admissions." And the assistant director and two members of the rescue team were upset that some medical staff said to clients whom rescue had just brought in for detoxification: "What, *you* here *again*?" During a general staff meeting on attitudes towards chronic repeaters, the antagonism between rescue team and medical staff became quite plain.

An incident which happened four years before the fieldwork period shows persistence of this built-in conflict. A staff member told the following story:

> Two rescue drivers brought in two candidates for detoxification. A corpsman examined both of them and said they did not need detoxification. The drivers protested to the director and assistant director, both of whom upheld the corpsman. Then instead of taking the two men to the shelter for the homeless or to the Metro City Alcoholism Clinic, the rescue team deposited them on the street in front of the offices housing the state alcoholism authority. The rescue team, the two men, or all four, presented themselves before the head of the authority and announced they had been denied detoxification at North Detox. The upshot was that North's director suspended both members of the rescue team for two days without pay.
>
> When asked for his version of the incident, the assistant director told more or less the same story. He went on to point out that rescue is supposed to bring in persons who are "candidates" for detoxification. Whether they get admitted or not,

however, is not the rescue team's decision. They are supposed to leave the admitting office and await the decision. If the person is not admitted, they are required to deliver him to a shelter or to the Metro City Alcoholism Clinic. Too many times, however, the team remains in the admitting office. The result of differing with orders is that the rescue team redefines the situation as a "personality conflict" rather than as an "issue." The assistant director went on to observe that if they are unwilling to just bring in candidates and not decide on their admission, they will lose their jobs.

The admitting office's 3 × 5 file listed all past and present clients. This card file sometimes had a "do not admit" after names of certain individuals. The "DNA" legend followed persons' names because they were considered "inappropriate referrals." This term connoted people who were psychotic, drug addicts, or who had medical problems the detox was not equipped to handle. Additionally, other individuals might have a "do not admit" after their names if they had been assaultive or verbally abusive in the past. There were, however, no clients who had been put on special restrictions or on therapeutic contracts. And, during the fieldwork period, most observed admission decisions were perfunctory, the screener deciding to admit or to refuse admission in a matter of minutes.

In addition, screening staff did not apply any of these restrictions on readmissions in a uniform manner at all. From time to time, staff felt a "fill the beds" pressure from "management"; the state alcoholism authority, which finances all public detoxes, reimburses detoxes according to their utilization rates. One medical aide commented that he did not appreciate the fact that sometimes nurses would readmit clients whose cards specified "do not admit" because of assaultive tendencies. And a detox technician, himself a recovered alcoholic, suggested that screening personnel who themselves were recovering alcoholics were more apt to be lenient in applying readmission criteria. Finally, North Detox, unlike most of the other detoxes, manifested many admissions conflicts coupled with persistent irresolution of these selfsame conflicts.

South Detox

Staff talk, observed screenings, and detox records showed that South Detox exercised more selectivity, where possible, over readmission of clients. South Detox's director said that the statewide association of 20 detox directors had commented negatively on South Detox's "restrictive policies." Their comment implied that South Detox was violating the "open admissions" norm. Observation of four different admissions revealed a variety of staff controls. In the first situation, a nurse talked at great length with a client who sought admission. This client had been detoxified a number of times previously at South Detox. The nurse told the client that his last admission had been under two special conditions; he had agreed to stay five days in the detox and to accept placement in a residential treatment facility on his discharge. Since the client had failed to keep up his end of the bargain, the nurse told him he was currently on a 90-day restriction. This meant that he could not be readmitted again at South Detox until the passage of 90 days. In the second situation, the assistant director took a call from a former client who sought to be admitted. Although there were empty beds at the time, the nurse on duty told the assistant director that she did not want that man coming in and gave no reasons for her decision. The assistant director then told the person on the phone that there were no empty beds in the detox and that he would have to try somewhere else. In the third situation, the admitting nurse (who at the time had only been working at the detox for some six months) wrestled with the problem of whether to admit a former client. A medical aide, himself a recovered alcoholic, talked her out of admitting the client, pointing out that alcoholics will say anything to get admitted but that this man could not be counted on to behave properly after admission. At first, she asked the aide, how was a person ever going to get a chance to get better if they were denied admission. Later, she thought it over and deferred to the aide's greater experience and refused admission to the candidate. The fourth situation involved the case of a client who had been admitted under a special agreement between himself and the medical person who screened him. The agreement was that he was to come in to be detoxified, to stay the minimum five days, and then to accept a post-detox referral placement that his counselor would work out with him during the period of his stay in detox. This client failed to keep the agreement, leaving two days after being admitted.

As a result, a staff member wrote down on his card in the 3×5 file that he was to be placed on a 30-day restriction. This restriction meant that he could not return to South Detox until 30 days had passed since this failure to keep the agreement.

Like most other detoxes, South Detox also had a 3 × 5 file listing the names on all past and present clients. Information on these cards included name, age, sex, religion, occupation, residence, dates of previous admissions and discharges, source of referral, and reasons for each discharge. "Inappropriate referrals" (psychotic, assaultive, drug addict, medical problems) had the "do not admit" designation appended. Specific security or therapeutic restrictions also appeared from time to time. Unlike most other detoxes, South Detox had a considerable number of cards in its file with specific 30-, 60-, and 90-day restrictions, and it was more apt to apply these criteria uniformly.

West Detox

Staff talked mainly about pressures to admit patients, black lists, against medical advice (AMA) discharges, and timing of admissions. A staff member said at a case conference that if a certain person presented himself at the detox, "we would have to take him." She said this after a counselor said that they could expect a certain client who had proven objectionable in the past to show up in a day or two, even though no one would want to admit this person. South Detox's director said that although public detoxes were not supposed to have "black lists," all of them did. A few staff members expressed concern over the number of clients who left AMA. And the admitting-clerk nurse, herself a recovered alcoholic, noted that a large percentage of admissions to South Detox took place late in the afternoon or early in the evening. Her explanation was that these clients were mainly concerned with getting as much drinking done as possible before thinking about shelter for the night.

South Detox records revealed more emphasis on inappropriate referrals and staff security than on therapeutic restrictions. Frequently, 3 × 5 cards would comment on the high frequency with which certain clients went AMA or less often, failed to stay five days. Evidence for variability in the application of detox admission criteria came from two sources—the records themselves and conversation with a patient. The South Detox Guidelines, a brochure for staff, states that ". . . a man should be drinking heavily for three days or more to need detoxification." It goes on to say that if a person had engaged in mild drinking for seven days and had been eating, that person may need drying out, but not detoxification. Information on all persons admitted during the two-months' baseline period showed at least ten who were admitted less than a day after their previous discharge from South Detox and almost two dozen who were readmitted seven or less days since their previous South Detox discharge. A South Detox client cites influences on staff decisions to readmit:

> The whole idea in a detox is to get you to take placement. I have signed out of here AMA a few times. In this area which is tough, there are a lot of trouble-makers. If a known trouble-maker comes to the door and rings the bell, they tell him there are no beds.
>
> Once in winter me and another guy with a leg in a cast were in a hallway making a lot of noise. The landlord called the police. The police came. They were on a hot call, so they dropped us off at the detox. Marty (a medical aide) came to the door. There were no empty beds but he let us sleep in the basement. We left in the morning.
>
> A lot of repeaters come here. As you probably know, they just stay for a night, maybe two. People get to know if a person is really hurting or whether he just wants a bed.

South Detox staff varied in applying readmission criteria. While there were few signs of staff conflict over readmissions, the detox director, Freddy F., said that there had always been a long-standing conflict between nurses and counselors at South Detox over admissions and discharges. In the past, he pointed out, counselors took the 5-day detox norm quite literally and would mark clients for discharge on their fifth day in detox without first checking with nurses to find out if they were medically well enough to leave.

East Detox

Much staff talk at East Detox dealt with premature discharges, staff reactions to them, and ways of coping with them. But, in turn, there was also considerable discussion of ways of modifying clients' long-term relationship with the detox as well as restricting contact with clients who refused to abide by staff rules.

One morning in the East Detox admitting office, Mac, a medical aide said:

> This morning was another plague. Only two people were supposed to go but actually eight left. (He went through the ad-

missions log pointing out the names of the people leaving
AMA.) Many of these AMA's go out the same day they come
in. All that work, then they leave. Sometimes it makes me so
mad, I could choke them.

And during an informal interview, Jean, an alcoholism counselor,
said:

> Monday is a bad day all around for everyone . . . The
> reason why Monday is hectic is that you come in and there are
> eight people waiting to see you. They want their clothes so
> they can go AMA. I've talked with Jackie O. (the detox direc-
> tor) about not working Mondays. Upstairs, one man is waiting
> to see someone about placement, while nursing staff is all up-
> set about all the people who are going AMA. They treat AMA
> like it was some kind of a crime. They really care, they're a
> very good, involved, first-rate nursing staff, and AMA's make
> them angry.

When asked about the people who come in, stay one or two days,
then leave AMA, Evelyn, a nurse said:

> They come in here when they're hurting, get a little treat-
> ment so they can go right back to drinking again. Some stay
> the five days or more only to end up doing the same thing. Lot
> of people come in and are just in and in and in. I think it must
> be quite frustrating for the counselors. At least I, as a nurse,
> can give them a pill.

A tape recorder in the admitting office had a printed notice under
it reading: "Tape all screening." Mac said people come in and
agree to do a number of things. A day or so later they deny ever
making any agreements. Now, he said, staff can play the tape back,
so clients can hear their own voice agreeing to staff terms. Later that
morning while Evelyn was screening Shane, Jean read him the
terms of his "contract." And that afternoon at the daily case conference, Jean said that Shane had "come in on a contract." Its terms
were that he was to go only when medical people said he was ready
to, that he was to participate in the program, and that he was to see
his assigned counselor. Two days later, Evelyn announced at the
case conference that Shane had left AMA and so he was now on a
90-day restriction.

An example of how counselors try to alter clients' relationships came up during a case conference.

> Peter (medical aide) popped in and said that a friend of Eddie D.'s called and said that he was bringing Eddie in and that he wanted to come in himself. Jean explained that she would see Eddie D. if he came in at 3:30. If he came in at 4:30, she would be gone. He could come in, but not his friend. The condition of his admission was that he would have to agree to sit down and talk about his drinking with his girl friend, Frannie F. who is already in the detox. When it turned out that Eddie D. and friend were planning to arrive at 4:30, Jean said she wouldn't be here and then repeated the conditions of admission. Jean said that Frannie F. cares for Eddie D. but not to the degree that he thinks. Meanwhile, Frannie F. lives with her sister who detests Eddie D. and the friends he brings around when drinking. Each blame their drinking on the other and that's what Jean wants to confront them with when they're together in the detox.

Admitting two clients to the detox who are friends can be a problem. Generally, staff fear that one friend may influence the other to leave the detox prematurely, usually to return to drinking together. One morning while screening two clients, Evelyn asked Mac to call West Detox to see if they had any empty beds. Later in the day she admitted both clients. Mac explained why she had him call West Detox. When she found out they weren't friends, she decided to admit both.

The nurse's ward book in the ICU contained a confidential list of some eighty names. One staff member referred to this alphabetical list as the "banned list," another as the "black list." Persons make this list if they are a relative of any current East Detox employee, an escaped prisoner, drug addict, psychotic, assaultive, or inappropriate medical referral. Temporary as well as permanent restrictions on readmission at East Detox have at least four different purposes. In the case of inappropriate referrals, the detox seeks to eliminate any future contact whatsoever. In the case of temporary restrictions as when a client breaks a contract, the detox seeks to stop subsequent detox-client contact for a stated interval, presumably as a kind of negative sanction. Two other kinds of restrictions, however, aim at either changing client behavior while in detox or after leaving it.

The field note excerpt below shows how temporary restrictions work.

> Taped to the fluorescent gray desk lamp on the table was a note about limit-setting for Nancy C. Joanne, a nurse, explained what the note meant: "Yesterday Nancy C., not too drunk, was in the examining room. Rather than permit me to examine her, she gave me a lot of shit. So I saw to it that she got her clothes. If she wants to get back in, she'll have to see me first."

Limit-setting tries to make clients more tractable during their time in detox. Restrictions, on the other hand, employ negative sanctions to get clients to make some small yet significant changes in their behavior after they have left the detox. This may be in keeping with the philosophy of Jackie O., East Detox's director. According to him, there are two types of clients: those who "use" the detox and those who enter into a long-term association with it. In his view, the detox has more success changing the second type.

Application of readmission policies at East Detox were most systematic. And, in turn, staff members neither disagreed with or countermanded any of these policies, whether temporary or permanent, during the course of the fieldwork.

Northeast Detox

Northeast Detox staff talked mostly about the kinds of troubles clients could make for them rather than on how they might help clients or work to alter clients' relationships with detox. They spoke of the legality of rejecting clients, admission contingencies, trustworthy and untrustworthy sources of referral, and clients under the ban.

Stanley, a corpsman who had been working at Northeast Detox for two months, commented on aspects of admission at Northeast as follows:

> There are only four patients here today. But I expect it to fill up real quick. Today is check day and people usually come in right after that. I think the place holds 25 and that there are beds upstairs. Guys want to come here, they sometimes wait at the Metro City Alcoholism Clinic even though they could go

somewhere else. It's well recommended. So I think that's a sign that it's a good place. Another thing I learned at a meeting last night is that though they come back, you can't turn them away. It's against the law. There's a state law which says you can't discriminate.

Admission contingencies include the number of sick patients already in the detox, number of staff on duty, and shift courtesy. As Jane, a nurse, pointed out, "the more people in the acute ward (eight beds), the fewer new admissions we can accept, and, the fewer people on duty, the fewer new admissions we can accept." As a demonstration of this point, one afternoon while there were still three empty beds in the acute ward, the assistant director, Grace W., came into the nurse's station and said that since the 4-12 corpsman had failed to show up for work, "admit no more patients." Ruth J., a nurse, exemplified shift courtesy one afternoon at 3:30 when the referral worker at the Metro City Alcoholism Clinic called her on the phone and asked if she had any empty beds and if she would accept a certain candidate he had in the Clinic office at that very moment. Since Ruth was going off duty at 4:00, she advised the worker to call back after 4:00, so that the nurse working the 4-12 shift could make the admission decision.

Bitter experience with some Metro City hospitals made screening personnel fearful Northeast Detox would become a "dumping ground." If some hospitals sent candidates for detoxification over without first medically clearing them, others were apt to refer psychotics, drug addicts, or persons with special medical complications which Northeast Detox was not prepared to handle. As a result, once nurses heard the name of the hospital calling them, they said they had no empty beds. Northeast Detox obtained many clients from the Metro City Alcoholism Clinic, where clients were medically cleared, before Clinic workers called up to ask about empty beds. As nurses became familiar with these workers, they came to trust their judgment in the case of first-time referrals.

On the other hand, in the case of clients seeking readmission, they referred to the "banned box." Sitting on a desk in the nurses' station was a 3 × 5 box with the legend "banned box" taped to the top. This box contained an estimated 300 file cards arranged alphabetically. Whenever a potential source of referral called, the nurse answering the phone would ask the name of the candidate, then ask the caller to hold the phone while she consulted the banned box. If the person's name appeared in the box, the nurse would usually say to the referring agent that she was sorry but there were no more beds available. If the caller was the Metro City Alcoholism Clinic worker, she was more likely to say the candidate was banned at Northeast Detox.

The following field note on the contents of the banned box gives some indication of the variety of troubles Northeast Detox staff have had with some of their clients:

> There are approximately 300 cards in the banned box. Some reasons for banning clients are: abusive, AMA's (too many), arson, assaultive, behavior problem, belligerent, destroys detox property, drinking on premises, drug user, escape artist, ETOH on breath, heroin use or user, kyloso (curvature of the spine), medical, management problem, polydrug addiction, pyromaniac, psychiatric problem, stabbed counselor, stole (either money or property from staff, patients, or both), threatening, etc.
>
> Sometimes there would be a note that the patient's file or record was missing or misplaced. Sometimes the ban would be because the person had drugs in him and the note said specifically that Dr. R. (attending physician) had ordered the ban. Bans are either permanent, indefinite, or for specific periods (30, 60, 90 days), or else they say that the person with the ban is to be evaluated or reevaluated on the problem that brought the ban in the first place when the client next presents himself or herself for readmission . . . Perhaps five times, a person was banned because he has a problem with females (staff, or, more often, patients). The ban might be highly specific as "do not admit when Linda S. is here" or "do not admit when there are female patients." Or the ban is general saying do not admit, has problem with females. In at least two instances the ban on particular patients was lifted by Andrew C., a counselor.

Most bans were for reasons of staff security or because clients were inappropriate referrals. Few of these bans were on therapeutic grounds. Jane E., a staff nurse, made some comments that suggest variability in application of readmission criteria:

> Northeast Detox's goal is to respond to people in crisis and to make them comfortable. Treatment for alcoholism comes

after they leave here in an outpatient clinic or a halfway house. Northeast Detox, from what I've heard has a low census but a high placement when compared with other detoxes . . . When people come in the same week, they might say to them that they obviously aren't being any help to them and that perhaps they ought to go to another detox. But *generally, they took the person back* (emphasis supplied).

Some three weeks later, Jane E. said she had admitted Donald L. under special conditions.

I just admitted Donald L. But, first, I made a special arrangement with him. I told him that he had to agree to stay five days and to take placement at the end of those five days or else I wouldn't admit him. He agreed. And, should he not stay five days this time, then I'll put him on a 90-day ban, *at least during the time when I'm on duty* (emphasis supplied).

Southwest Detox

Staff talked at Southwest Detox about AMA's, restrictions on readmissions, and characteristics of "regulars." Again, much like staff at some of the other detoxes, staff seemed somewhat more concerned with reducing contact with clients who really didn't want help or who were coming back too often.

Southwest Detox drew many clients from the Metro City Hospital Alcoholism Clinic. This comes about for one of two reasons. First, most Metro City chronic inebriates knew that the Clinic was the place to go if they needed detoxification. Although a person might have to sit in the Clinic for a couple of hours or more, in time a bed at one of Metro City's six public detoxes would ultimately become available. Secondly, if persons call West, Northeast, or Southwest Detoxes, and have never been detoxified there, the nurse or admission clerk (in the case of Southwest Detox), will notify the caller that they or the person for whom they're calling for must first go to the MCHAC first to get medically cleared.

Over time then, clients become known to Southwest (as they do of course to all the other detoxes). Thus, when a client or his representative calls Southwest Detox to find out if a bed is available, the admission clerk first puts the caller on hold (unless she recognizes the name, the voice, or both) and checks the 3 × 5 file to see if the person has been in Southwest Detox before and if there is a "hold" on the person. If the person is known to Southwest and there is no "hold" on him, then the admissions clerk will tell the caller to come to the detox and that they will hold the bed for two hours. Ralph H., a medical aide who doubled as admissions clerk, explained the phone-call system as follows:

> When someone calls up, I have to look up the records to see if the person has been here before, and if so, is there a hold on him or her. (What's a hold?) They like for a person to stay five days. If a person leaves before five days, that's called AMA or "against medical advice." Now if a person does that, then he or she can't come back for at least five days. Or sometimes, it's for longer. And, sometimes after they meet upstairs, they take the person off the "hold."

In the screening that Southwest Detox personnel do over the phone, they ask a lot of questions. Often they will ask the caller (if the person is acting as a referral agent), "does he know it's a five-day stay?" or "will he stay five days?" In most detoxes, a five-day stay separates acceptable from less acceptable clients. At Southwest Detox, it became an explicit basis for moral evaluation of detox clients.

Ralph H. said he had seen some clients a few times since he's been working here. He called them the "regulars" because quite a few of them were coming every five days or so, particularly during the winter. Vera S., an administrative assistant, voiced the typical detox staff misgivings about clients who came back fairly regularly.

> The idea of providing shelter for someone who needs it is right. But sometimes I wonder whether we're accomplishing anything. I sometimes get discouraged seeing the same people coming back. Some of them really don't want to do anything about their problem.

At Southwest Detox, staff made use of both an admissions log notebook as well as the 3 × 5 client file. "Do not admit" or simple "DNA" appeared after many names in these records, which included brief descriptions of inappropriate referrals and the like. More often, DNA would be coupled with a 30, 60, or 90-day restriction. Staff placed these restrictions on clients when they left AMA too many times. These records reveal staff concern about security.

And, similarly, they show impatience with inappropriate referrals. But, mainly staff restricts readmissions to punish clients for failure to comply with staff's five-day norm. Such modification in future behavior staff might seek from these clients would be that on their return they would have to comply with staff length-of-stay norms if they wished to remain in good standing and to be assured of continued services. And, at least in the short run, Southwest Detox staff would not have to make contact with clients who seemed guilty of being unwilling or unable to use treatment services in the approved manner.

Unlike other detoxes, Southwest Detox had few staff conflicts over readmissions problems and a systematic procedure for resolving such conflicts as did occur. For a person to get on the "do not admit" list, they would have to "do something." If a client did something, staff wrote up an incident report. At the Thursday staff meeting they discussed the report. Then the detox director (at the time, Earl S.) decided whether or not a person's name went on the list. These restrictions were permanent, indefinite, or for the usual fixed time-periods of 30, 60, and 90 days. At subsequent staff meetings "holds" were reevaluated, and again, the detox director decided if any of them were to be removed.

Variability in applying admissions policies exists, of course, because staff exercise discretion. Southwest's staff did not apply admissions criteria uniformly as the following comments of Dot E., admissions clerk, and Maureen J., head nurse, reveal.

Dot E.: There's been a lot of AMA's today. I wouldn't have let them in. They haven't finished their drinking. I know it sounds hard, but they're not sick enough. You let them in like that, and in a little while they say, where's my money, where's my clothes, I want to get out of this dump.

Maureen J. (an hour later): You should have been here yesterday. We had 14 admissions. Vera S. was on. She took them all. Dot E. wouldn't have. (Seven of these 14 admissions left AMA.)

The previous summaries give some idea of how detoxes try to solve problems of readmissions and retention. Each of the detoxes define, interpret, and respond to these problems in somewhat different ways. These responses cumulate into what is called here staff culture. All of the detoxes from time to time emphasize different aspects of the readmissions and retention problems. In addition to these changes, there are the stable aspects which make it possible to differentiate between detoxes and their cultures. Thus, all pay close attention to matters of staff security though some are more vigilant on these matters than others. In turn, all need to respond to matters of organizational survival; nonetheless, it was only the staff at North Detox and Northeast Detox which talked about empty beds and the need to fill them with clients. And with regard to continuing relations with those clients who tend to return, the detoxes could cut off contacts with such clients permanently or for fairly long stretches of time. And so far as manipulating contacts with clients, they could have short-term or long-term goals in mind. They could be concerned with making clients less troublesome during their stay in detox or they could see if they could maneuver clients into a durable association in which staff both pointed to and assisted in achieving some measurable changes in behavior and attitude over a long period of time.

Selective emphases in these matters or lack of them help to characterize the six detoxes. Thus, Northeast Detox showed the least concern over readmissions or retention, the most on matters of staff security. Southwest Detox applied strict controls, when possible, on clients who failed to stay five days or who left AMA. South Detox combined controls on restriction and retention, with more emphasis on changing behavior in detox than afterwards. East emphasized after-detox somewhat more than in-detox. West Detox evinced more concern about retention than restriction. And North Detox, judging from staff talk on the two subjects, was as concerned with restriction as with retention. What both of these detoxes shared in common was great concern with readmissions problems coupled with erratic application of readmission criteria.

Table 1 gives some indication of how well the various staff cultures solved the problem of readmissions. It does so by comparing and contrasting both the length of stays and percentages of readmissions in the six detoxes.

Inspection of the table shows that South Detox retains clients much longer than any of the other detoxes. On the other side, Northeast Detox ranks the lowest in retention with an average of only 2.9 days, at the same time that it has the highest percentage of readmissions of all. East and Southwest were near the top with identical length of stay averages of 3.5 days apiece whereas North and West were closer to the bottom with identical average lengths of stay of

3.2 days. Southwest, East, and South have much lower percentages of readmissions than do Northeast and West. Thus, the table lends support to the notion that ways of coping with detox problems along with client characteristics need to be taken into account when considering relations between process and outcome.

THE PROBLEM OF CHANGING DETOX CLIENTS

Public detoxes, like all human service organizations, have multiple goals. They seek to shelter, save lives, maintain if not improve physical health, detoxify, and rehabilitate. Rehabilitation, hardest to achieve, stands at the top of the goal hierarchy. Detox counselors work with clients on recovery. Recovery from alcoholism means making personal changes. Counselors cannot make those changes for their clients. They can only assist them in the process. Again, detoxes may vary in how they arrange matters for initiating changes in the lives of their clients.

Counseling arrangements in detoxes consist of an ethic and a structure. Ethic refers to approaches counselors take when contacting clients. Structure includes external aspects which may affect these contacts in some way. External aspects include counselor-client ratio, alcoholic-non-alcoholic counselor ratio, frequency of medical staff contacts, and frequency of staff meetings. The detox summaries which follow point up these differences in counseling arrangements. After these summaries, an examination of their influence on clients follows.

North Detox

North Detox, largest of the detoxes, had four counselors. Two recovered alcoholics took an AA approach with clients while the other two were more eclectic. The ratio of counselors was 1:14, largest caseload of them all. During field work there were two detox staff meetings: one was a training session, while the other dealt with staff attitudes towards readmissions. Case conferences took place every afternoon. At these conferences, medical staff, usually the floor nurse or corpsman, reported on the medical status of the clients (number of days in detox, medication, medical complaints, etc.). Assigned counselors would generally say after the name, ''he's mine,'' ''haven't seen yet,'' ''is going OP Friday,'' ''he's

Table 1. Length of Stay and Percentage of Readmissions by Detox

Detox	Length of Stay (in days)	Percentage of * Readmissions **
North	3.2	---
South	4.1	37%
West	3.2	43%
East	3.5	33%
Northeast	2.9	53%
Southwest	3.5	31%

*   Based on the number of clients readmitted to each detox during two-month's baseline period.

** No data available on North Detox readmissions during baseline period.

playing games,'' or the like. Counselors would be present for the entire meeting, whereas medical staff would come in and leave by floors when they had finished reporting on clients on their floors. Medical aides did not attend these conferences. Staff reported information on clients in summary fashion. This made it possible for medical and counseling staff to share information on all clients currently in residence in 15 or 20 minutes. These conferences sometimes helped medical staff to see clients through counselors' eyes just as counselors sometimes came to see clients through the eyes of medical staff. A nurse might say, for example, that she thought a certain client was motivated and might profit from talking with a counselor. In turn, a counselor might say that a certain client still seemed too "jiggy" (tremulous) to talk to a counselor. There were few signs of disagreement or conflict between the medical staff and the counselors.

Because of readmissions, counselors became quite familiar with many clients. Thus, they could usually tell at a glance when just stopping by the bed of a newly readmitted client on "day one" whether the person wanted to talk with them on the following day. For the most part, clients wanted to talk with a counselor only if they sought "placement" after detox. If they had no intentions of seeking placement after detox, then counselors had no more contacts with them.

South Detox

Both South Detox counselors were recovered alcoholics. One, a woman who had regained her sobriety in Alcoholics Anonymous, followed very closely the ideas about alcoholism that she had acquired through her membership in the famous fellowship. She felt that unless persons with drinking problems affiliated with Alcoholics Anonymous, their chances of sobriety were slim. A black man was the other counselor. He had regained his sobriety while living alone in a single room by attending regular meetings with a social worker in one of the state's outpatient alcoholism clinics. More eclectic about recovering from alcoholism than his staff partner, he might tell his story in resource meetings but was always careful to point out that people should pick out what they thought might work for them in recovering from alcoholism.

The ratio of counselors to clients at South Detox was 1:10. South did not have daily case conferences where counselors and medical staff reviewed clients' progress. But it held more general staff meetings than all other detoxes. Most of these were held daily. Some of these meetings were followed by special case presentations, at which a consultant might be present to aid in subsequent discussion. Others were case presentations where counselors would present cases of clients with unique problems to the assembled staff (including medical aides). The idea seemed to be that someone on the staff might be able to suggest a new approach. At the close of one of these meetings, one counselor said that although new ideas had come forth, he felt good after airing his feelings.

West Detox

A man and a woman served as alcoholism counselors at West Detox. Both were recovered alcoholics and "staunch AA's." Both followed the AA approach although they were somewhat sympathetic to alternate ways of becoming abstinent. The ratio of counselors to clients was 1:10. Daily case conferences on the progress of clients took place in a small office. At most of the other detoxes, clients were assigned to counselors as they came in. But at West Detox, counselors volunteered, usually saying "I'll take him." None of these conferences lasted longer than fifteen minutes and a good deal of the conversation centered around the health of the client, degree of deterioration, strength of motivation to give up drinking, and the like.

The woman counselor said it was quite hard to reach "educated" clients with the message of AA because they found it "too simple." The male counselor criticized detox counselors who thought they were doing rehabilitation counseling, which he argued, could not be done in a detox. He thought five days insufficient, ten-day stays being more to the point. He said his work with clients had three phases: crisis-intervention, confrontation, and referral.

The director of West Detox was a recovered alcoholic who had sobered up in a Metro City halfway house and had also joined AA. Later, he worked as an alcoholism counselor at East Detox before he became director of West Detox. He was most critical of his two counselors. According to him, the male was bigoted, sexist, overbearing, insensitive to clients and their feelings, and all together too insistent on AA. The female, he felt, was limited by her inability to get to work on time and her over-reliance on the AA message. Only one staff meeting was held at West Detox. That one was solely for the purpose of introducing the researcher to the staff. Unlike most of the other detoxes, West Detox had meetings for clients both in the morning and in the afternoon. These meetings consisted of "rap sessions," films, slide shows, and resource presentations. AA meetings were scheduled nightly.

East Detox

East Detox had three alcoholism counselors, two women and one man. One of the women was both a recovered alcoholic and a member of AA; the other two counselors were not. East Detox had the lowest counselor-client ratio of the six detoxes, namely 1:7. Working relations seemed pleasant and counselors seemed bent on helping clients with all of their life-problems rather than insist they solve their "booze problem" first. Two staff meetings took place during the field work at East Detox. Case conferences took place daily, averaged an hour in length, included medical aides, and showed great diversity and variety of comments on clients, their problems, and their prospects. These East Detox case conferences suggested that staff took director's philosophy quite seriously. This philosophy called for helping clients to make little changes in their lives rather than enormous ones such as giving up drinking permanently upon discharge.

Northeast Detox

As noted earlier, Northeast Detox was situated in a fairly large black neighborhood. At the time of field work, only one staff member, a female nurse, was white. The rest of detox staff was black. Both alcoholism counselors, one a male, the other female, were recovered alcoholics as well. The counselor-client ratio was 1:10. Both had sobered up in halfway houses. Shirley B. had regained her sobriety through affiliation with Alcoholics Anonymous; Andrew C. has become abstinent through residence in a halfway house for black alcoholics which had its own group approach to personal change. Northeast's counseling ethic mixed values. However, the alcohol education program at Northeast Detox seemed somewhat attenuated. During the field work, staff showed two movies to clients, and one halfway house resource meeting occurred. But no general staff meetings or case conferences took place.

Southwest Detox

Both counselors at Southwest Detox were brothers and members of Alcoholics Anonymous. Both started, at different times, as medical aides and, in time, worked themselves up to become counselors. Both pushed AA as the best way for alcoholics to solve their drinking problems. The younger of the two counselors had decorated his small office with a collection of AA symbols, insignia, and slogans. Similarly, Southwest Detox was supposed to have an AA meeting every night of the week. On the other hand no case conferences between medical staff and counselors took place nor were there any general staff meetings held during the field work period.

The ethnographic summaries of counseling arrangements at the six detoxes have sketched in variations in detox approaches to the task of influencing clients. These sketches make it possible to compare and contrast patterns of counseling and then to assess their influences. For example, they suggest that public detoxes follow one of two ethics. Either they "push AA" or they pursue a more eclectic approach. With regard to the structure of their counseling arrangements, they have heavy, moderate, or small caseloads, while their counseling staffs are either completely or partly made up of recovering alcoholics. When it comes to contacts counselors make with medical staff, these detoxes range from those with daily and long case conferences through infrequent and short case conferences all the way to no case conferences whatsoever. And, similarly, with respect to meetings of the whole detox staff, they may have many, few, or no such meetings at all.

What kinds of influence do these counseling arrangements have upon their clients, if at all? How, if at all, does process affect outcome? Measures of output may help to answer these questions. The present exploration focuses on specific measures of detox output. Making the detox the unit of analysis, rather than individual clients, this study compares the three kinds of discharges the six detoxes compiled during the two-months' baseline period. Just as there are several routes into detox, so are there different ways of leaving. The percentages of TP, OP, and AMA discharges may differentiate one detox from another.

Table 2 below lists discharges and percentages at the six detoxes.

Table 2 suggests possible relationships between counseling arrangements and detox output. Thus, for example, Northeast Detox which had an eclectic ethic coupled with minimal counseling structure obtained the most TP discharges, along with the second highest percentage of OP discharges and the second lowest percentage of AMA discharges. Similarly, East Detox with an eclectic ethic and maximal counseling structure obtained the highest percentage of OP discharges, the second highest percentage of TP discharges, and the lowest percentage of AMA discharges. By way of contrast, South-

Table 2. Kinds of Discharges by Detoxes

Kinds of Discharges

Detoxes	OP	AMA	TP	Total Admissions
North	49%	38%	13%	706
South	49%	37%	14%	301
West	44%	41%	15%	356
East	67%	17%	16%	320
Northeast	54%	20%	26%	277
Southwest	30%	55%	15%	324
				2284

west Detox, with a "push AA" ethic and a minimal structure produced the highest percentage of AMA discharges and the lowest percentage of OP discharges. West Detox with a similar ethic and comparable structure achieved the second highest percentage of AMA discharges. North and South, on the other hand, with eclectic ethics and comparable structure obtained almost identical percentages of all three discharges.

A TYPOLOGY OF DETOXES

These results, by no means definitive, suggest a typology of detoxes. This typology may help to better understand detox operations as well as to suggest policy changes. A cross-classification of the way detoxes manage readmissions with their counseling arrangements yields four types. On the one hand, detoxes can be strict or lenient in the ways they manage readmissions; on the other they may have either routine or adjustive counseling arrangements. Strict detoxes have clear readmissions policies, systematic procedures for resolving staff disagreements on readmissions, and fairly uniform application of readmission criteria. Lenient detoxes have readmissions policies which, whether clear or unclear, get inconsistent application, coupled with much staff disagreement, little resolution. Similarly, adjustive counseling arrangements include an eclectic along with optimum structure. Routine counseling arrangements encompass a "push AA ethic" with either too much or too little structure. The six detoxes in the present study fit this typology approximately in the following ways.

1. *Strict-routine.* Southwest Detox monitored readmissions strictly, confined counseling almost exclusively to its two AA-oriented counselors. As a result, it attained a fairly high length of stay (3.5 days) coupled with the lowest percentage of readmissions. At the same time, it topped all detoxes with 55% AMA discharges. "Push AA" programs often generate strong counterreactions. As one client said while waiting to be screened in one of the detoxes: "There's nothing worse than having someone push AA on you when you're coming off a drunk." A study of two public detoxes found similarly that the AMA rate varies directly with "staff fervor for AA methods" (Regier, 94:1979).

2. *Strict-adjustive.* South Detox exemplifies the strictest controls on readmission, including a strong emphasis upon retention, with an

adjustive counseling pattern. The result was that it had the highest length of stay of all six detoxes (4.1 days) and stood third in percentage of readmissions. Its retention rate is all the more remarkable since it served almost the identical clientele that North Detox did. East's high production of preferred detox outcomes, as noted above, derives in part from its admissions policies as well as its adjustive counseling, characterized by its favorable counselor-client ratio and its system of intensive case conferences.

3. *Lenient-routine.* West and North Detox were quite similar in lax applications of readmission criteria, staff disagreements, and absence of any system for resolving staff conflicts over admissions. While West "pushed AA" and North was more eclectic, the counseling structure in both resulted in routine contacts between counselors and clients. West had the second highest percentage of AMA discharges. In general, its output and North's were almost identical.

4. *Lenient-adjustive.* Northeast had a pattern of admission policies that bordered on laxity while its counseling was eclectic in ethic, minimal in structure. In consequence, it achieved a paradoxical output record. It had the shortest length of stay, the highest readmissions rate, the highest percentage of TP's, the second highest percentage of OP's, and the second lowest percentage of AMA's.

SOME POLICY IMPLICATIONS

In coping with recurrent problems detoxes evolve a set of ways for dealing with these problems. This staff culture, obviously an historical product, can change under certain circumstances. Consequently, fitting the detox to its type can well suggest a set of policy implications. This paper now concludes with some suggestions for how changes in policy may help staff to deal more effectively with their problems and, in the bargain, to improve their output.

Detoxes which may be experiencing persistent conflict over admissions might profit by combining the examples of South, East, and Southwest. Such a combination would include a clear policy on readmissions and retention devoted to changing client behavior both in and after detox, a system for adjudicating and resolving admissions conflicts coupled with a pattern of general staff meetings which would sustain staff consensus by frequent communications on policy.

Similarly, for detoxes with lenient policies of readmissions, institution of behavioral contracting with so-called "chronic repeaters" might well establish a set of attainable and measurable goals that both staff and client can work towards. This, perhaps more than anything else, would reduce the high level of unwarranted staff expectations which in the opinion of Jackie O. and others is the principal explanation for staff burnout among detox staffs. A last policy implication concerns the shift from routine to adjustive counseling patterns. The "push AA" approach works best with those clients who least need it while it tends to alienate those who might well profit from a softer sell. The rare AA member who has a "slip" and who comes into detox knows full well how to get and to stay sober and will most likely reaffiliate with AA just as soon as he is discharged from detox. By contrast, typical chronic public inebriates may well profit more from a synthesis of an eclectic ethic and high structure.

SUMMARY AND CONCLUSIONS

The main explanation for why public detoxes have not achieved the goals alcoholism policy reformers projected for them resides in the characteristics-of-clients argument. Broader understanding of detox operations requires the addition of cultural analysis. This paper has attempted to do that by showing that what goes on between staff and clients in detox needs to be included for a fuller understanding of detox operations and treatment outcomes. In coming to terms with built-in organizational dilemmas, detox staff used available organizational resources to cope with key problems of readmission, retention, counseling, and policy conflicts. The principal organizational resource they came to draw upon was the fund of collective experience gained through working with varieties of detox clients. This fund, from which they all drew, was their particular staff culture. If some detoxes developed a fund which centered around changing clients, a few focused upon sustaining clients. And a few others were content to settle for simply processing clients.

REFERENCES

Annis, H. M. and Smart, R. G. Arrests, Readmissions, and Treatment Following Release from Detoxification Centers. *Journal of Studies on Alcohol,* 1978, 39, 1276-1283.
Fagan, R. W., Jr. and Mauss, A. L. Padding the Revolving Door: An Initial Assessment of

the Uniform Alcoholism and Intoxication Treatment Act in Practice. *Social Problems*, 1978, 26, 232-246.

DenHartog, G. L. *"A Decade of Detox": Development of Non-Hospital Approaches to Alcohol Detoxification—A Review of the Literature*. Jefferson City, Missouri: Missouri Division of Alcohol and Drug Abuse, June 1982.

Daggett, L. R. and Rolde, E. J. Decriminalization of Public Drunkenness: The Response of Suburban Police. *Archives of General Psychiatry*, 1977, 34, 937-941.

Regier, M. C., *Social Policy in Action. Perspectives on the Implementation of Alcoholism Reform*. Lexington: Heath, 1979.

Rodin, M. B., Pickup, L., Morton, D. R., and Keatinge, C., Gimme Shelter: Ethnographic Perspectives on Skid Row Inebriates in Detoxification Centers (this volume).

Shire, J. and Smith, J. Drying Out: An Exploratory Study of Staff in an Alcoholic Detoxification Unit. *Annals of the New York Academy of Sciences*, 1976, 272-273, 409-419.

Udell, B. and Hornstra, Good Patients and Bad: Therapeutic Assets and Liabilities. *Archives of General Psychiatry*, 1975, 34, 1533-1537.

Westermeyer, J. and Lang, G. Ethnic Differences in Use of Alcoholism Facilities. *International Journal of the Addictions*, 1975, 10, 513-520.

Experiences of Incarcerated Alcoholics: Chronic Drunkenness Offenders in a County Workhouse

Florence Kellner Andrews

INTRODUCTION

Chronic drunkenness offenders are men whose conditions and activities have constituted a persistent law-enforcement problem in America since the middle of the 19th century (Rooney, 1970). Aside from their propensity to be addicted to alcohol, a deficit of conventional social ties to families and jobs and their lack of permanent shelter have rendered attempts at rehabilitation to be more problematic than would be the case if alcoholism were the only complication. Studies of the homeless man, the disaffiliated man, or the chronic drunkenness offender attest to the very high recidivism rates for this type of person (e.g., Pittman and Gordon, 1958; Rubington, 1962; Zax, Gardner, and Hart, 1961) and the improbability of most programs directed toward sobriety or change in life-style having any appreciable effects upon their drinking habits, other activities, or living conditions. This type of arrestee is subject to the ''revolving door'' phenomenon—a perpetual arrest, release, and rearrest pattern which seems to be consistent across the United States.

Probably because drunkenness offenders are so resistant to change, are frequently arrested for minor criminal offenses (e.g., public drunkenness, disorderly conduct), and are familiar to police and judges, the activities involved in arresting and sentencing them often violate accepted legal procedure: they are rounded-up quickly, held until trial, and adjudicated in a matter of minutes (Wiseman, 1970; Bahr, 1973). Aside from the contradiction to acceptable procedures involved in the criminal processing of the police case inebriate, the legality of the application of criminal proceedings to

Florence Kellner Andrews, Department of Sociology and Anthropology, Carleton University, Ottawa, Canada K1S 5B6.

these cases has been seriously questioned. Since 1966, when two decisions of the Federal Court declared it to be unconstitutional to convict alcoholics for displaying their disease symptoms (Driver, 1969), there have been efforts to decriminalize offenses involving public drunkenness (Pastor, 1978; National Institute on Alcohol Abuse and Alcoholism, 1977), and decriminalization has occurred in a number of places. Alternatives to correctional establishments for the handling of homeless inebriates have proliferated during the past 20 years. These structures—primarily halfway houses and detoxification centers—have had mixed results in terms of rehabilitation, humane treatment, and effective control of public inebriates.

The following account describes an organization which evolved to accommodate the needs and characteristics of homeless inebriates and focuses upon the relationship between the correctional officers and the chronic drunkenness offenders. Unlike the situations of the homeless inebriate described by Wiseman (1970) and Spradley (1970) the men discussed here did not make systematic rounds of social agencies, missions, and jails; nor did they languish in "drunk tanks" with very poor facilities. Although a number of county establishments provided incidental services to these homeless men, the County Workhouse had the most consistent and enduring association with them. This association, described below, resulted in mutual satisfaction of both the chronic offender and Workhouse personnel. This establishment is a correctional facility; therefore, rehabilitation had low priority. However, given the present state of knowledge of alcohol addiction and the present state of resources available for dealing with the difficult combination of homelessness, drunkenness, and disaffiliation, it is believed that this situation provides an example of a viable and beneficent response to the problem of drunkenness offenders.

SETTING AND METHODS

Midstate County Workhouse* is located within a major metropolitan area on the American Northeast coast. It belongs to the "house of corrections" category of incarcerating institutions (Fox, 1972). These establishments are administered by counties and are concentrated in the older, colonial areas of the United States. The Work-

---

*The name of the Workhouse is fictitious, people's names are also pseudonymous.

house was built in the middle of the 18th Century as a result of State legislation giving county officials power to construct a combination almshouse for the relief of the "deserving" poor and a poorhouse for the incarceration of vagabonds and petty criminals (Rothman, 1971). Designed in the traditional style of the post-medieval European workhouse, most inmates slept and spent their time inside the house in a large wing, an open space with no dividers between the beds.

Persons convicted of misdemeanors sentenced for 364 days or less served their time in the Workhouse, including those sentenced for offenses involving public drunkenness. Sentences for these offenders were typically for 30, 60, or 90 days. Although the sentences were short, as sentences go, many drunkenness offenders spent more time incarcerated than they did outside, frequently returning to the Workhouse for another conviction within a month after release. During the time of the research, drunkenness offenders constituted about a third of the 90 to 100 male inmate population. Other inmates in the Workhouse were people convicted of other misdemeanors (e.g., fraud, some traffic offenses, and petty theft). Just prior to the research time, people charged with felonies were put "on hold" in the Workhouse until their trials. About a third of the inmate population was on hold, and the presence of alleged felons necessitated alterations in a security system which was typically quite relaxed. Tighter surveillance was imposed upon the "holds," and because of the presence of holds, the security system for the entire Workhouse population was becoming more stringent.

The Workhouse is situated in a municipality containing mainly farms and suburban residences. Access to the establishment is from a minor, but well-travelled, State route. The main building of the Workhouse is set behind numerous acres of farmland which belong to the institution. From the outside, the place resembles a farm, more than it does a correctional institution. There are neither gates nor fences nor any other barriers separating the Workhouse grounds from the land surrounding them. Other structures on this County property include a farmhouse, a poultry shed, the warden's house, a building with offices for The Inmate Welfare Society,* and a

---

*This agency provided some medical aid to incarcerated inmates, arranged for payment of equipment such as glasses, dental plates, and crutches, and attempted to place released inmates in half-way houses and jobs upon release. Release placement for chronic inebriates was almost invariably unsuccessful, because they broke house rules through drunkenness and failed to hold a job for more than a week or two.

maintenance building, with supplies and tools for the upkeep of the buildings, vehicles, and farm machinery. The organization was responsible for much of its own maintenance, and the farm provided produce and poultry for consumption by Workhouse residents and other county establishments, such as the jail and hospitals. Research at the Workhouse was conducted during 84 visits over a 14 month period. Data consist of fieldnotes from observation and interviews with 61 inmates and 17 staff members. All interviews were of the focused, open-ended type. Inmate interviews contained topics regarding life in the Workhouse, views of other inmates, and views of the staff. The inmate interviews ranged from twenty minutes to an hour and a half, most of these being about forty-five minutes. Staff interviews usually lasted over an hour and included a variety of job-related topics, such as recruitment, work satisfaction, views of inmates and staff, routine, and security measures. All interviews were conducted in complete privacy. Short notes were taken during the interviews and the complete conversations were reproduced at a typewriter, with the aid of the notes and memory, usually on the same day the interview took place. Likewise, fieldnotes were typed up during the same day as a Workhouse visit. Thirty of the inmates who were interviewed could be classified as chronic drunkenness offenders, having had more than three arrests for drunkenness-related offenses within a year and a half. Their ages ranged from 35 to 72, with fairly even distribution in the 40s, 50s, and 60s. None of these chronic inebriates were living with families; although some had been married and had children, very few had any contact with either their ex-spouse or their children.

LIFE IN THE WORKHOUSE

"Treatment" for Alcoholism

About thirty inmates in the population at any one time consisted of people with drinking problems. Of these, any of them might suffer an alcohol-withdrawal attack a few days after being incarcerated. Local hospitals, both public and private, refused to admit inmates undergoing delirium tremens. Because of the lack of availability of outside help, Workhouse personnel instituted a fairly effective routine for dealing with withdrawal. Diagnosis was based upon familiarity with particular repeaters and recognition of an array of symptoms commonly associated with alcoholic withdrawal. If a man were known to have had DT's during a previous sentence, he was watched especially carefully.

From fieldnotes, Day 55: Lieutenant Walsh talked to inmate Mike Angus (an inebriate regular) asking how he was. Angus came to the window saying he was fine, but that it had been rough for awhile (he'd just come out of DT's). I asked Walsh how he knew when DT's were coming on. Walsh said you could not tell except when they set in. Also, they know to watch a guy who has been here before and who had them already. With Angus, Walsh said, you could not tell. He was shaking when they brought him in—his hands were shaking. "So we put him in the small wing and he was alright for two days. Then, he gives me this piece of paper, telling me to be careful of it and to put it aside for him. Nothing was written on it, so then I knew."

Fieldnotes, Day 37: An officer recalled a number of years ago when he went to a cell to check on a guy who seemed to be out of the rams (delirium tremens). "We wore grey shirts then." He was sitting there calmly and the officer asked him how he felt. Said he was fine and looked at the officer's shirt and asked (seriously) when he started driving Greyhound buses.

Treatment for withdrawal routinely involved the administration of sedatives, isolation, and special surveillance of the withdrawing inmate until the DT's subsided.

Fieldnotes, Day 39: I asked the sergeant what they do for someone who has gone into DT's. He said, "Only thing we can do is to put them in a cell and remove everything from it but a mattress so they don't hurt themselves. We try to force drugs down them if we can. Too bad about the hospitals. They don't take them; they don't want them."

"What would happen if you actually brought them to a hospital?" I asked.

"I remember trying to get them in. They would give them back to us."

"Which hospitals have you tried?"

"All of them . . ." (the sergeant named 4 hospitals in the area).

There were times when people in DT's did get brought to the hospitals, and this was when convulsions were frequent or when an inmate did not seem to be coming out of withdrawal as soon as the staff thought he should. Although a physician visited the Workhouse for an hour or two every weekday morning, inmates' withdrawals were rarely timed to coincide with the doctor's presence. Despite the lack of medical training or sophisticated facilities, the Workhouse staff handled the alcoholic problems with substantial competence and no little concern for the inmate/patient.

Other Aids to the Chronic Drunkenness Offender

Aside from dealing with the medical problems of the alcoholic inmate, the staff actively expressed concern for the well-being of these inmates regarding other aspects of their lives. The chronic drunkenness offender was the type of inmate for which the physical and formal structure of the Workhouse was most appropriate. Moreover, these inmates were necessary to the maintenance of the establishment. Because they were not escape risks, they could be assigned to various work crews—the farm, the kitchen, poultry tending, repairs, and grounds (landscaping)—with minimum concern for security and surveillance on the part of the staff. A typical day for the chronic offender involved an early breakfast followed by "sickcall"; three hours' work; lunch; three hours' work; "freetime" (wash-up, cards, talk, TV); dinner; "freetime"; and "lightsout". Being more-or-less regular residents of the Workhouse, these inmates were familiar with their jobs, the Workhouse routine, and the rules. The dependability of the chronic drunkenness offenders in doing their assignments and in not causing trouble, along with a familiarity with them based upon long-term association, were appreciated by the staff; and this appreciation was demonstrated in several ways.

When chronic inebriates or regulars were released, there was some attention to their immediate comfort. Although transportation rules dictated that released inmates be driven to the County seat, staff on transportation duty took the men to their particular locales. The County provided no pay to inmates for work done in the Workhouse. Many of the drunkenness offenders received some income through pension checks, veteran's disability allowances, or welfare money, but they were often without cash when they were released. Correctional officers frequently gave a man a small amount of their own money to take care of immediate needs. Sometimes, officers arranged for jobs for these men, but became discouraged, because few were known to have kept a job for any appreciable time. Staff members were concerned enough with regular inmates to expend considerable effort helping some of them when they had problems in or outside the institution. If an inmate needed a new set of false teeth or glasses, officers contacted the appropriate agencies; guards made considerable effort to make certain that temporarily disabled chronic offenders had shelter during release time; and there were instances of guards' smuggling in alcoholic beverages for these inmates. Officers were also kown to be passively permissive: they "looked the other way" when these inmates managed to obtain whiskey through friends' smuggling it onto the Workhouse grounds.

The Chronic Offender's Time in the Workhouse

Most of the men with alcohol-related offenses were consistent, although not constant, residents of the Workhouse, spending a total of about a half a year incarcerated and the other half outside, with several months between sentences. About 10 of these chronic inebriates claimed the Workhouse as a permanent residence (their pension checks and other correspondences were addressed to them in care of the institution). These men typically stayed outside the institution less than two weeks between 90 day sentences and often refused to take advantage of "good-time," (time taken off sentences for good behavior), preferring to complete their entire sentences.

As was mentioned above, the taking on of holds affected the lives of the sentenced inmates, because of a general tightening-up of security measures and the imposition of stricter disciplinary procedures for both officers and inmates. From accounts of the way life was before holds are incarcerated there, it was evident that a considerable degree of behavior which is considered unconventional for a correctional establishment could be tolerated without the sacrifice of internal order. Notes from an interview with an inmate:

MacFadden told me about how guards used to bring in booze all the time here, and make a small profit on it. It has not been coming in since last summer, however. I asked if that was because of the three guards who got fired because of smuggling. MacFadden said yes, ". . . and maybe that scared the others" (other guards). "Which others?" Williams and Hunt used to smuggle regularly. I asked how the inmates had the money to pay them. Family and friends used to make a drop. It is easy to make a drop here if you know the lay of the land. For instance, you tell your visitor to come Tuesday morning and to leave a package or an amount of money in a small bag attached to a string and put this in the dried-up well by the warden's old house. "You know he is going to make the drop Tuesday AM, so you get there in the afternoon. Used to be done all the time." There was this guy who used to have it good and used to supply all the others with beer. There is Parson Lake out a ways behind the pumphouse,* and his wife used to rent a row-boat and row up with a case of it. He used to get in the boat and the two of them would polish off half the case out on the lake— this was summertime, of course. Then, he would give the other half to the rest of the pumphouse gang.**

Even though security was tightened for all inmates, the people who were the Workhouse regulars remained on good terms with the officers, expressed an understanding of the difficulties of their work situation, and some of these repeaters even expressed some loyalty to the place, affection for the guards, and pride in the work they did on their assignments. The following quotations from inmate inter-views should provide some examples of the quality of their relation-ships with the corrections officers and their attitudes toward being in the Workhouse.

> Inmate: You have some guys here—we call them floaters—
> they go to jail in other places sometimes. They keep
> saying to us, "My, God, this sure beats Glenville or
> Estmont!" They say that. We have the best food
> here.
>
> Interviewer: Have you been in any other places?
>
> Inmate: Oh, sure, in Virginia, in Washington, in Connecticut
> . . . but this is the country club of them all . . . Oh,
> the food is better than any other place I or most of the
> guys have been in. And the trust they have in you—
> that's good, too.

---

*Shed with maintenance equipment.
**Inmate maintenance crew.

Interviewer: How does trust come into it?

Inmate: We are let outside and nobody is on our back all day. This is a good thing. They don't hound you. It's a damn good shelter, too. In the winter, when the cold gets so much you can't take it anymore, you go up to the railroad station and find a bench for yourself and stretch out. Soon, the railroad cop sees you, and boom!, here you are.

Many of the regular inmates knew that they were indispensable to the smooth running of the place—that not many people could do the jobs that the Workhouse officials depended upon the regulars to do.

Inmate: This ain't bad. I do minor repairs here. I'm on the chicken gang. Just the other day, this guy driving the truck smashed those big feed boxes flat. Now you can't tell me he didn't see them. Flattened them right out. I fixed them so you wouldn't know they were broke. That's what I do. Fix everything that's broke.

*   *   *

Inmate: I have the feeling someone is dropping the dime on me.

Interviewer: What's that mean?

Inmate: Well, this cop comes to me and tells me he's been told to pick me up. How does that sit when I'm not doing anything wrong? He come up and says, "I'm told to pick you up." I have a feeling the deputy warden calls in when they are having trouble with the turkeys, because I'm their turkey tender. I always get picked up in the fall or late summer, when the turkeys are young.

Interviewer: Why you?

Inmate: I make them live. They die easily. Look how does it look to you? I get picked up September 14 this year, and there are all the turkeys, just born. November 26 I get out. Half of them are killed at Thanksgiving and the other half at Christmas . . . I know turkeys. I had three years of agriculture in high school. You have to

know when to feed them . . . feed them quietly, and
don't scare them. And Riley (poultry supervisor),
what does he do? Sit on his big pooper and count the
chickens.

The relationship with the staff was one which at least entailed recognition of authority, if not absolute respect. There was a sense of
"fair play" among the inmate regulars in their relationships to the
guards. That is, if a party does what is expected of him, he is entitled to have his expectations filled as well. Similarly, the very least
a man is entitled to is not to be hurt or bothered, granted he does not
hurt or bother other people (Gouldner, 1960). These quotations
from inmate interviews express this view of inmate and guard reciprocity.

Inmate: I haven't seen an officer here yet give a guy a hard
time if he acts right.

Inmate: Never had any trouble with no guards. That is, unless
you hand them a lot of gup. They do the best they can
do.

Inmate: They (the guards) are good to you, to tell you the
truth, and help you when they can. If you are friend-
ly, so are they. They don't bother you. Talk nice to
you.

Inmate: I figure it's just like in the service; you treat them
with respect and they treat you with respect. You see,
I did learn something in the service.

With the exception of occasional misunderstandings which are
present in any social group, the interchange between the chronic offenders and the guards was smooth, predictable, mostly informal,
and often quite satisfying to both guards and inmates. Even the occasional breaking of regulations by these inmates was tolerated by
some of the guards, although less outright violation was permitted
since the presence of holds increased to noticeable and disturbing
proportions. This is not to say that most of the regulars were
perfectly happy with their life situations of repeated incarceration.
Older men who had been inmates in the Workhouse for many years
tended to accept the place as being as close to a home as they could

reasonably expect. People who were at earlier stages of "going on the skids" were more inclined to hold some hopes of being able to break the revolving door cycle. Until they did, however, this place was not "half bad."

CONCLUSIONS

Claims to the success of a social program depends, in a large part, upon the criteria employed to define success. Although we cannot assert that the Workhouse provided either treatment for alcoholism or social rehabilitation in the conventional sense, we may claim that this organization has achieved a viable accommodation to the chronic police case inebriate which is at least superior to most accounts of agency-drunkenness offender relations in the literature.

As far as treatment for alcoholism goes, the Workhouse afforded an opportunity for sustained sobriety, shelter, and food. While there were occasions for drinking at the Workhouse, abstinence from alcohol was the rule, and opportunities to drink occurred very infrequently. Detoxification for a month or more, combined with a good diet and substantial activity probably contributed much to the physical well-being of these men. Even among the older Workhouse inmates, there was no evidence of marked physical or mental deterioration apparent to this investigator. This is not to say that there was no room for improvement, especially as far as treatment for withdrawal was concerned, but, given the facilities available, withdrawal occurred with a minimum of mishap.

While there was little in the way of efforts directed at rehabilitation available at the Workhouse, there was also little in the way of punishment. The temporary loss of freedom was accepted by the men as a condition of the lives they chose and as a fair exchange for the relief from coping for survival "on the street." In addition to food and shelter, activity on the work gangs provided opportunity to socialize and militated against the boredom usually associated with incarceration. The work activities the drunkenness offenders engaged in at the institution generated both a degree of self-respect and a sense of responsibility. Although feelings of pride and responsibility may have little to do with recovery from alcoholism or social rehabilitation, we may assume that people are happier with these feelings than without them.

It is, perhaps, irreverent to suggest that some people who do not desire rehabilitative services should not have such programs forced upon them. The issue of decriminalization makes such force more likely, or, depending upon the resources available in the community, results in short-term detoxification and little relief from the exigencies of homelessness. Chronic drunkenness offenders often neither want nor benefit from the activities of agencies which attempt to cure alcoholism or to effect their integration into mainstream society. At the same time, some intervention is necessary in order to control the factors of public nuisance and to allay the deteriorative effects of alcohol dependence and homelessness.

The Workhouse situation provides an example of a workable compromise for this type of alcohol addict who has little or no conventional support systems and, often, has little motivation (at least, for the present time) to change his way of life very much. While treatment and social recovery programs were not available at the Workhouse, forced incarceration enabled these individuals to recover physically and to take advantage of the social welfare programs in the community when they were released. A few chose to do so, with some success; a few kept trying; many of the drunkenness offenders intended to ''straighten out'' sometime in the future. Until that future comes, the presence of the Workhouse leaves that option open.

REFERENCES

Bahr, H. M., *Skid Row: An Introduction to Disaffiliation,* New York: Oxford University Press, 1973.

Driver, R. J., "The United States Supreme Court and the Chronic Drunkenness Offender," *Quarterly Journal of Studies on Alcohol,* 1969, 30, 1:165-172.

Fox, V., *Introduction to Corrections,* Englewood Cliffs, N.J.: Prentice-Hall, 1972.

Gouldner, A., "The Norm of Reciprocity: A Preliminary Statement," *American Sociological Review,* 1960, 25:161-178.

National Institute on Alcohol Abuse and Alcoholism, First Special Report to the U.S. Congress on Alcohol and Health. Washington, D.C., U.S. Government Printing Office, 1971.

Pastor, D. A., Jr., "Mobilization in Public Drunkenness Control: A Comparison of Legal and Medical Approaches," *Social Problems,* 1978, 25:4.

Pittman, D. J. and W. T. Gordon, *Revolving Door: A Study of the Chronic Police Case Inebriate,* Glencoe: Free Press, 1958.

Rooney, J. F., "Societal Forces and the Unattached Male: An Historical Review," in H. M. Bahr (ed.), *Disaffiliated Man,* Toronto: University of Toronto Press, 1970, pp. 13-38.

Rothman, D. J., *The Discovery of the Asylum,* Toronto: Little Brown and Co, 1971.

Rubington, E., " 'Failure' as a Heavy Drinker: The Case of the Chronic Drunkenness Offender" in *Society, Culture, and Drinking Patterns,* D. J. Pittman and C. R. Snyder (eds.), New York: John Wiley and Sons, 1962, 146-153.

Spradley, J. P., *You Owe Yourself a Drunk: An Ethnography of Urban Nomads*, Boston: Little, Brown and Co, 1970.

Wiseman, J., *Stations of the Lost: The Treatment of Skid Row Alcoholics*, New York: Prentice-Hall, 1970.

Zax, M., E. A. Gardner, and W. T. Hart, "Public Intoxication in Rochester: A Survey of Individuals Charged During 1961," *Quarterly Journal Studies on Alcohol*, 1964, 25:660-678.

A Case of Ideology in Alcoholism Treatment

Melvin Tremper, Ph.D.

ABSTRACT. This is a description of the response made by the staff of an alcoholism treatment program to the strains of their work roles. The strains included multiple lines of authority, low professional status, and conflicting role demands. The staff coped with these strains through use of a treatment ideology. This ideology selectively emphasized those elements of alcoholism treatment approaches which served to reduce the strains experienced by the staff. The staff was able to construct an ideology because alcoholism treatment had not yet developed an empirically verified treatment technology. It is speculated that when such a technology is developed treatment staff will have to find other ways to reduce the strains experienced in their work.

This paper is based on field observations in an inpatient alcoholism treatment unit for men which combined detoxification and rehabilitation services. It's primary focus is on how the treatment staff of the unit utilized the therapeutic concepts of "dependency" and "motivation" as part of a treatment ideology which allowed them to cope with the strains of their work roles.

SETTING

The alcoholism treatment unit was part of a state mental hospital in the Eastern United States. The hospital was located in a rural setting remote from major highways and 15 miles from the nearest public transportation. It consisted of several 40-50 bed brick "cottages", some larger patient units, an administration building, a medical building, and living quarters for many of the hospital staff, scattered about several acres of rolling meadows.

Melvin Tremper, State of Maine Office of Alcoholism and Drug Abuse Prevention.

The unit itself consisted of a 12 bed detox ward comprising one floor of the medical building, and a 40 bed rehab unit housed in one of the cottages. Although the unit comprised only about 10% of the total beds, its 450 annual admissions accounted for 30-35% of the hospital's annual total.

The unit was administered by a part-time psychiatrist who also had primary clinical responsibility for the unit. Other clinical duties were handled by a full-time psychiatric resident, various psychiatrists in training on a rotating basis, two social workers, a part-time physician, a psychologist and around the clock nurses or nurse's aides.

I originally entered the unit in order to study the clients as part of a larger research effort focused on the treatment patterns of chronic public inebriates in the state. While collecting client data, I observed the staff's behavior and their treatment ideology. I became fascinated by the language the staff used to describe both their own behavior and that of the clients. Their perceptions of the events on the unit were quite different from both mine and the clients. I stayed on the unit for two years, eventually collecting client information only to provide a reason to stay on the unit and observe the staff.

SOURCES OF STRAIN

As I became more familiar with the difficulties faced by the staff in carrying out their professional duties, their perceptions of events began to take on meaning. These perceptions were shaped by a more or less coherent treatment ideology which acted to protect the staff from the strains they encountered in working on the unit.

These strains arose from two major areas. One was the size and nature of the client population. The second was the organizational structure of the unit itself. The fact that the clients being treated were alcoholics was in itself a source of strain. Being engaged in the treatment of alcoholics is not a high prestige pursuit. Whatever the merits of the position that alcoholism is a disease, there are strong elements of moral and social condemnation of alcoholism still present in our society. Drama contains images of the weak willed, whining alcoholic, comedians portray the silly, sloppy drunk. Alcoholics in the street are a cause for concern for the public order and the sanitation of the urban scene. Alcoholics on the job are covered over until they function so badly they are fired. Alcoholic mothers are a source of shame for their husbands and children alike.

The stigma of alcoholism in part rubs off on those who treat them. Partly because of this and partly because the treatment of alcoholism is still viewed as less successful than the treatment of other conditions, the treatment of alcoholism is often professionally unrewarding. Wechsler and Rohman (1982) have recently reported "A substantial number of students, social work and counseling students in particular, expressed a reluctance to become involved in the treatment of people with alcohol-related problems" (p. 953).

Like other client groups, the alcoholic population differs within itself in many socioeconomic characteristics. These differences impact on treatment providers in two ways. In the first place, client characteristics affect the prestige of the persons providing treatment. The higher the class of the clients being treated, the higher the prestige of the treatment providers. In the second place, client characteristics often have an effect on the client's responsiveness to treatment. This relationship is particularly true in the alcoholism treatment field. Outcome studies have shown that clients with lower incomes, longer drinking histories, fewer family supports and community ties, (including a steady job) are less likely to become treatment successes than those with opposite characteristics.

Many of the clients at the unit were from the less prestigious and harder to treat segments of the client population. Thirty seven percent had not graduated from high school, 44% came from unskilled or semi-skilled occupations, 55% were married and living with their wives, and an estmated 20-25% were unemployed at the time of admission.

The large proportion of lower class clients was largely the result of the unit's status as the only state operated inpatient alcoholism treatment program in the state. While limited alternative treatment resources were available for those with money, there were none for those without. For this reason, the unit was the last resort for many referral sources as well.

The larger study of treatment patterns in the state mentioned earlier revealed that some referral sources saw the unit as a "dumping ground" for problem clients. The staff was aware of this, and was frustrated at bearing such a label. The pattern of readmissions, and the continual receipt of feedback that former clients had returned to drinking further demoralized the staff.

Formally, the staff could do nothing to alter the situation since the unit was compelled by law to admit clients in need of treatment. A section of state law specifically required this institution within the state's mental hospital system to "... admit, retain, and provide care and treatment for ... alcoholics ... who require hospital care ... subject to availability of facilities for hospitalization and treatment thereof". Thus, formally, the staff had no discretion concerning the admission of clients appearing for treatment.

This legal mandate is part of what I call the organizational structure of the unit. Yet another aspect of the unit's structure was its relationship to two state government bureaucracies. Although the unit was part of a mental hospital and was thus under the jurisdiction of the state Department of Institutions and Agencies; it was partially funded by, and also under the jurisdiction of, the state Department of Health which was the parent agency of the Division of Alcoholism Control. The mental health system expected the unit to respond to the administrative needs of the hospital of which it was a part and to serve the alcoholism treatment needs of the entire state mental hospital system. This meant not only providing services for clients referred by other hospitals within the system, but also preserving a "mental health approach" to the entire area of alcoholism treatment. The foundation of this approach was that alcoholism was a manifestation of other, underlying, mental illnesses.

The Division of Alcoholism Control operated a small system of outpatient counseling services throughout the state. It sought to use the unit as a resource for clients for whom outpatient counseling was not appropriate. Many of the outpatient counselors themselves tried to use the unit as a place to send clients who had no other place to live. Unit staff were continuously urged to attend statewide meetings held by the Division, and were expected to work closely with the outpatient counselors on mutual clients.

These demands were sometimes conflicting, sometimes overlapping. In any case they created an area of ambiguity regarding the true role of the unit.

Multiple allegiances and conflicting demands are also found within the structure of the unit itself. This extends to the authority structure of the cottage, and the allocation of staff's duties.

As described above the unit was headed by a part-time psychiatrist. Dr. Z., the incumbent at the time of the study, had held the position for a decade. He had control over admission, treatment and discharge decisions regarding individual clients as well as overall program structure. Since he only worked part-time, he was not always available when important decisions had to be made. Nominally, the psychiatric resident was in charge at these times.

However, the short term nature of their assignments reduced their ability to act decisively.

A total of four social workers filled the 2 positions during the time of the study. Only one had a masters degree. They all viewed their positions on the unit as a way station to something else. The nursing attendant staff had many years experience on the unit. They told Dr. Z. what they thought he should know, and ran the daily unit routine. Formally, the social workers outranked the attendants. However, by virtue of their experience and the fact that they were often the only medical personnel on site, the attendants would overrule the social worker's plans and schedules for client meetings.

All members of the staff, from administrator to attendant, are subject to multiple authorities. For example, the social workers are under the authority of the head of the unit, the Addictions Unit social work supervisor, and the hospital social work supervisor. The nursing staff is subject to the head of the unit, the Addictions Unit nursing supervisor, and the medical officer of the cottage. The staff also has to satisfy hospital-wide administrative and record keeping demands.

In addition to demands generated by persons within the hospital, the social workers must face demands made by persons outside the hospital. These demands come from prospective patients, the families of both prospective and current patients, and professionals outside the hospital. On the one hand, there are those professionals who are interested in getting a client of theirs admitted to the hospital, or who are interested in the welfare of a client already in the hospital. On the other hand, there are those professionals whom the social workers must use as resource persons to effectively carry out post-discharge plans for patients. These categories of professionals are not mutually exclusive, so it is necessary to please referees in order to have resources for future referrals.

Of course satisfying the demands of external agents is more than just a device to make the social worker's task easier, for the social workers are acting as the unit's representatives to these external agents. Any disruption of relations with these agents may seriously interfere with the unit's functioning insofar as this functioning depends on external agents for referrals to postdischarge facilities. The demands of the patients must be dealt with in the context of all these other demands.

The attendants suffer from a similar set of conflicting demands.

In addition, they are relatively powerless to actively satisfy patient demands. In most cases, they can only act as ombudsmen mediating between the patients and others. For example, the attendants receive many requests for medications and/or treatment. They cannot honor these requests without first consulting with a physician. In addition to being asked to perform services directly, the attendants are also asked by the patients to request services from other members of the staff. In fact, since Dr. Z. is generally unavailable to the patients, a large proportion of all patient requests consist of asking the attendants to ask Dr. Z. if a certain action is allowable. The attendants are also asked to seek action from the social workers and from other segments of the hospital bureaucracy. None of these others appreciate being bothered with constant requests for action, medication, and special treatment of all sorts. The attendants are aware of this and are reluctant to bother them. Therefore, patient requests are a source of trouble for the attendants.

Within this context of conflicting demands, there are several factors which serve to promote client demands on staff.

There are social factors inherent in the situation of being hospitalized which induce patients to act dependently. These factors include both the normative expectations of the patient role in American society at large and the specific structural requirements of the institution itself.

On the most general level lie the cultural norms in our society regarding the role of the sick person. Probably the best known exposition is by Parsons (1958) who has suggested that the role of the sick person is analogous to that of the child. Neither is expected to function as a fully adequate adult. Not only is the sick person excused from his normal responsibilities, he is also expected to become dependent on others for care.

The hospitalized patient is even more dependent; he is isolated from all his normal resources and much of his personal autonomy must be sacrificed to the requirements of efficient hospital management. The fact of hospitalization forces the patient to accept the sick role, and an extreme version of it at that. Minor illnesses may be treated at home or in a doctor's office, the more serious ones require hospitalization, hence the hospital patient is more ill. It would seem that this would act to increase the pressures toward dependency.

The patients at the alcoholism treatment unit viewed admission to the cottage as an indication of more serious illness. Interviews with patients on the medical ward who had not yet been admitted to the cottage showed that some completely misunderstood the criteria for selection. They believed that cottage admission was limited to those in a more deteriorated condition, who "really needed treatment", when in fact the more seriously ill were screened out. While their assumption was erroneous, it was not unreasonable in light of the common societal views of the functions of hospitals and more specific pieces of information which prospective patients glean about this unit.

The image of the hospital as a place to go to be taken care of is presented to the patients by many referral sources. Quite naturally nonprofessionals, such as Alcoholics Anonymous (AA) members, see the hospital as a place to receive help. Prospective patients are told "you can get help at the hospital". The implication is that the patient will passively receive benefits from attending the hospital.

Thus the societal image of the hospital as a place for receiving help is reinforced by messages from referral agents. This message is repeated when the patient arrives at the hospital. His first hospital experience is an interview with a social worker, in which the social worker invariably explains his function as that of a helping agent. The patient is told the social worker is there to help with any problems he may have with the outside world during his hospitalization. He is actively encouraged to call on the social worker for aid. And during the course of this interview the patients are told "What the program has to offer you."

So far we have seen that the sick person is expected to behave relatively passively; that patients are expected to be even more passive; that many patients see admission to the unit as an indication of severe illness with its implied passivity; and that even if a patient were still to believe he should be an active agent, he is told by referral agents and unit staff that the unit is a place in which he will be taken care of. These are, after all, only expectations and implications. Perhaps a truly independent personality type would be able to ignore them and behave independently. However, there is more within this situation than expectations of dependence; there are also structural features requiring it.

Although, unlike many mental patients, these patients are allowed to maintain a stock of personal possessions, there are still limitations on them. For good reason they are not allowed to possess any drugs. However, since this ban applies to such drugs as aspirin, cough drops and the like, the patients must either suffer pains and discomfort or go on "sick call". Having to minister to a daily quota of minor complaints could well create the impression that the patients were just like complaining juveniles. Another restriction is that the men are not allowed to possess more than three dollars in cash. If they are admitted with more than this on their person, the rest is either put into an account at the business office or may be used to purchase a limited number of "books"—sets of coupons good at the patient store. In order to buy a book, the patient must go to a staff member and apply for one, then after a few days the book arrives and is given by the staff member to the patient. Since the cottage staff have no real control over how long it takes the request to be sent to the business office, processed and returned, they often become annoyed with the patients' persistent inquiries about when they will receive their books. Obtaining money from the account at the business office must also be done through the social workers at the cottage who take a form, typed in triplicate, to the business office and physically receive the money and bring it back for the patients. This is a bothersome task for not only does it consume time which the social workers might be devoting to other duties, it reduces them to mere errand boys. Cashing a check, unless it is a postal money order, also requires the assistance of the social worker and the business office and again takes several days.

In addition to these relatively minor dependencies the patients must rely on the social workers for guidance in the bureaucratic jungle of insurance forms, welfare payments, job hunting and other areas. Many of the regulations are obscure and complicated, many of the forms ambiguous. Well-educated patients find them difficult enough to cope with. When it comes to those with minimal education, professional help is a necessity. Even if a patient were to have adequate knowledge of the proper procedures, his relative isolation in the hospital would make it difficult to perform his own social services. Incoming and outgoing mail is slow, patients are allowed out of the cottage to use pay phones only at certain times of the day, and, to my knowledge, no patient has ever been allowed to receive an incoming call. Thus, even if in only a physical sense, patients are dependent upon social service help. When it is considered that some patients face the prospect of leaving the hospital with no money, no place to stay, no family and no job, it is understandable that they will seek aid from the social workers.

The point of describing these difficulties is to demonstrate that the staff is faced with a set of role demands which exceeds their capacity to satisfy them. This is not a reflection upon the staff's capacity, but on the nature of the demands. Not only is the total demand rather large; there is also occasional conflict between different demands. In short, the staff is in a setting conductive to what Goode calls "role strain". Viewing role relations as transactions wherein role players attempt to minimize costs and maximize rewards, Goode declares ". . . ego perceives and responds to alter's power positions" (p. 487).

THE STAFF'S SOLUTION

As with other role players, the social workers would prefer to allocate their resources to satisfy the demands of the more powerful members of their role set. In this case, the most powerful role partner is the head of the cottage. He is followed by the various administrative and professional personnel within and without the hospital. Last, and definitely least, are persons seeking admission to the hospital. Somewhat above them are patients already within the hospital.

The expedient path to maximum rewards would appear to lie in the direction of slighting the demands from patients in favor of those from more powerful groups. This path is made somewhat harder to follow by the existence of a set of professional ethics (e.g., Moore, 1970) and a formal job description which direct the social workers to give maximum attention to the needs of the patients. Although the attendants are not part of a truly professional group, they, too, feel an obligation to serve the patients.

The social worker's dilemma extends beyond a conflict between expediency and ethics. The patients are not the only role partners whose claims are legitimate. The claims of both administrative superiors and professional colleagues also have legitimacy. This tripartite allegiance to institution, profession and client, is a feature of several other occupational groups, notably physicians and college instructors. Despite the frequency with which such a dilemma occurs, there is no institutionalized mechanism for allocating priorities among the competing claims. It is true that professional ethics require service to the client. It is also true that institutional structures require compliance with directives.

The choice between these sets of legitimate demands is often dictated by the following considerations. First, compliance with institutional rules can be justified by claiming that, in the long run, a smoothly functioning organization is best for the patients. Second, institutional demands are usually made in reference to visible measures of production. This leads to a tendency for workers to focus on performing the more visible elements of their task. For example, staff members would be more likely to complete required paper work rather than converse with a patient. Third, in the typical case, compliance with institutional directives is the alternative most likely to be tangibly rewarded. Intangible rewards such as approval can also flow from both the administration and from one's fellow workers whose jobs may be made easier by compliance with institutional demands. This would induce staff members to comply with institutional requirements. It could also lead them to focus on guiding the patients to act in such a way that the task of fulfilling institutional requirements was made easier. For example, Malone, Berkowitz and Klein (1962) found that in their client contacts, nurses tended to focus on those aspects of care which, if not done, would considerably inconvenience the department (e.g., meeting diagnostic appointments). Thus, whatever legitimate reasons there may be for such compliance, it often gives the appearance of pure expediency.

It is suggested here that in order to reduce the confict between the ethical requirements to satisfy the patient's demands and the practical requirements to satisfy the more powerful role partners, the staff have resorted to defining many of the patients' demands as illegitimate—that is, they have defined the patients as over-demanding and over-dependent. Not only does the staff define many of the patients' demands as illegitimate, but they also claim that meeting these demands is untherapeutic since it serves to reinforce the dependent behavior. Thus the concept of dependency offers a convenient and professional vocabulary to justify not meeting all the patients' demands.

The concept of motivation was used by the staff in a similar way to provide the staff with a means of coping with the strains caused by the unit's unique position in the state's treatment system. It also provided the staff with an explanation for treatment failures.

As described above, the unit operated under the jurisdiction of two separate segments of the state bureaucracy. In addition, it was virtually the only referral resource available to many social service agencies, as well as desparate individuals throughout the state.

This affected the unit staff in two ways. First, the total potential demand for the unit's services far exceeded its capacity to provide them. Second, the majority of the clients referred to the unit were low in prestige and low in expected success rate. In systems theory, every system seeks to maintain a boundary between it and its environment. A key to maintaining that boundary is the ability to control the inputs received from the environment. If the unit is seen as a system, then a major "input" consists of the clients admitted to the unit. Controlling the number of clients reduces the burden on staff members and allows them to devote more time to effectively treat those who are admitted. During the two years I observed the unit, the detox was occasionally filled to capacity but the rehab unit was never full. In fact, there were rarely more than 30 clients there at a time.

Controlling the type of client admitted is also important. It conserves that unit's resources by admitting only those clients who may potentially benefit from the treatment. It reduces the number of potentially discontented clients who may exert a negative influence on the morale of the unit and the operation of group therapy sessions. In addition to these therapeutically based reasons, it also allows the staff to select "congenial" clients who may be more pleasant to work with.

The staff maintained control over admissions in two ways. The first was to violate the letter, if not the spirit, of the law and simply deny admission to a client. The second was to institute a two-stage admission process where clients were first admitted to detox and then screened for admission to rehab.

Ironically, the first option was used most often on clients who may have needed treatment the most—those who were intoxicated. Intoxicated clients were often brought by "lay professionals", that is ministers, sheriffs, probation officers, or active AA members, or by concerned family members. The staff viewed such episodes as attempts to "dump" clients on them. They saw such clients as "merely" in need of medical treatment, which although provided by the unit, was not its primary purpose. They reasoned that intoxicated clients were not rationally motivated for treatment and thus could be denied admission.

The head of the unit occasionally admonished the staff for such behavior indicating that it was far safer to admit such clients and "turn them out at staff". "Staff" in this sense was a screening session during which it was decided if a client should be admitted to rehab from the detox unit.

During a staffing, clinical staff discussed the client's case history and then the client himself was presented for an interview. Often, prior to the client's appearance, the staff decided that the client was unsuitable or "unmotivated" for admission. They would agree upon this beforehand and further agree that they would try to get the client to indicate that he did not want treatment, or wanted to seek it elsewhere. By having the client himself refuse treatment, the staff escaped the provision of the law requiring admission to those who sought it.

The concept of motivation was the key to control over admissions. This concept was an important part of the staff's conceptual framework which views the clients as persons who are unable to control their drinking. This lack of control is attributed to underlying emotional difficulties. The client's use of alcohol is seen as an ineffective substitute for a realistic solution of his life problems. Not only is the alcohol ineffective in solving problems, its use in this manner creates more problems. Physical treatment of the effects of acute intoxication is viewed simply as a means to prepare the patient for actual therapy. Proper treatment is conceived of as using group therapy to aid the patient in achieving insight into his faulty life patterns. To achieve this insight, the patient must take an active part in the treatment program. There are two main goals to the treatment. One is to bring about total abstinence; the other is to help the patient resolve his underlying emotional difficulties. In the long run, the former depends on the latter.

The concept of motivation acquires significance within this treatment framework. For, if this treatment modality is to be effective, the client must first recognize that he has a problem with alcohol and that he must seek help in dealing with this problem. The staff emphasizes that it is not possible to effect a "passive cure", that is, one without the client's own active involvement in the treatment process. In short, the client must have a commitment to achieve sobriety. Such a client is said to be "motivated".

This description of the staff's framework was constructed from numerous observations and interviews. Despite, or indeed, perhaps because of, the concept's central importance to the staff, there was no clear-cut definition of it. Attempted definitions were given less in terms of abstract conceptualizations than in terms of referring to concrete attributes of patients. The following is excerpted from the field notes of a conversation with a staff member in which I specifically asked her to define the concept for me.

Q. What does motivation mean?

R. (Quizzical look.)

Q. Could you give me a definition in twenty-five words or less?

R. (Silence, apparently thinking.) That's hard to say.

Q. Well if it's that hard, maybe you could just give me some indication of what you would look for in a patient, what you would call a motivated patient.

R. A number of things. Alertness, awareness, and what kind of person he thought he was.

Q. What do you mean by that?

R. Well, how he saw himself in a group or as an individual. If somebody was too detached like a schizophrenic, he wouldn't be too good. Then there's involvement. Some men can talk up a storm and it sounds real great but when it comes to action you don't see much. They have to be involved with their problem. Then there's the way they move their hands and body.

Q. What?

R. Yes, you've seen them in staff, the ones that sit there like a dead fish, unless they're in a depression which I could understand; they don't seem interested. When you get involved you move your hands to emphasize a point. You don't just sit there doing nothing. And of course there's what brought him here. If he comes of his own accord, that's one thing, if he was pushed into it, that's another. Then there's how he arrived. If he was dumped off in the middle of the night all drunked up . . .

Q. It doesn't sound easy.

R. It isn't. Of course if he isn't motivated for treatment here, that doesn't mean that he isn't motivated to get treatment some other place like AA or somewhere.

Q. Then a guy may be motivated to stop drinking but just not motivated to get treatment?

R. Yes. Then there's fear. If there's too much fear that's not too good. Apprehension is understandable but if the motivation is just some great fear, once that's removed the er . . . . (shrugs)

Q. (After an interruption by others walking by.) Then a guy could be motivated to stop drinking but still not motivated to come to this place?

R. Yes. This place requires a more active approach. The man must be willing to give some effort to help himself not just sit there passively like at some places.

(Further interruptions ended the discussion here.)

These remarks show that the key to motivation is whether the patient is "willing to give some effort to help himself." They also show that there are many indications of the presence of motivation. While these indications are logically related to the staff's conception of alcoholism and its proper treatment, they are also useful to the staff in maintaining autonomy vis à vis external agencies and in selecting "congenial" patients whom the staff will find more pleasant to treat.

Take for example the importance attached to the method of contacting the unit utilized by the patients. A patient who makes the initial contact with the unit himself is seen as more motivated than one who has been assisted by some other—for example, his wife. Patients who are brought to the unit in an intoxicated condition are seen as having little motivation. One staff member spoke disparagingly of the quality of the patients who are "dumped off in the middle of the night", presumably at the whim of others.

It is possible that desire for treatment is associated with the mode of entry to treatment. However, other factors such as the client's physical condition and interpersonal skills, and his involvement with other agencies are also related. Clients who don't need immediate detoxification with resources and social support can call the unit in advance and make an appointment for admission. Clients who are in poor physical condition and who are lacking in resources and support are more difficult to treat. They are also likely to contact the unit in ways which are defined as indicative of low motivation. Clients who are brought to the unit without warning by outside agents are seen as lacking in motivation. By defining these clients as unmotivated and unsuitable for admission, the unit staff is able to convert their need for organizational control over the admissions process into a therapeutic issue. Although they can't control external agencies, they can insulate themselves from many of their demands. Ostensibly, only information concerning the client's motivation was relevant in formulating admissions decisions. Yet, observations of admission staff indicated that certain formally irrelevant characteristics seemed to be associated with the attribution of motivation. Patients who were young, neat, well-dressed, articulate and charming, were more likely to be certified as motivated than those who lacked these characteristics. Some of these characteristics were explicitly recognized by the staff as playing a role in the admission decision. Artriculateness is one such characteristic. Its role was formally justified on therapeutic grounds. The ability to sustain a coherent conversation does more than make a client pleasant to talk to. It is evidence that he can effectively participate in the group therapy sessions which play a major role in the treatment process. The importance of age was also occasionally explicitly recognized and formally justified. It was considered better to treat younger clients since they could contribute more productive years to society.

Most of these secondary characteristics were not given explicit recognition despite the role they played in the admission decision. The characteristics on which patients were judged suitable for admission constituted the staff's concept of the ideal patient. Such a concept is not unique to this unit. As Ryan (1971) observed: "The average patient is an interesting, reasonably cultured and well educated person, rather attractive, and an enjoyable conversationalist. This complex of characteristics is summed up by the psychodynamic concept 'well motivated' " (p. 143).

There is some evidence that such patients were desirable not only because they were more pleasant to work with, but also because such patients were seen as evidence of the worth of the unit itself. In the staff's ideology, the motivated patient was the ideal patient; that is, the one most likely to benefit from therapy. In actual practice, the ideal patient; that is, the one most likely to benefit the therapist, was defined as motivated. Justifying the choice of congenial patients was one of the functions of the concept of motivation.

The staff of the unit was faced with a variety of strains and problems. While they lacked the power or authority to change the conditions which created these strains, they were able to reduce the impact of the strains on themselves by creating an ideology. The staff's response contained two essential elements. The first was to define all elements of the treatment situation in therapeutic terms. The second was to selectively focus on a therapeutic approach which reduced the staff's workload and increased their autonomy from external demands.

CONCLUSIONS

Creating a "treatment ideology" to suit staff and organizational needs is not unique to this unit. A decade of experience with a variety of substance abuse treatment programs in Maine has presented me with an equal variety of treatment ideologies. Nor is it unique to alcoholism treatment. An example from a related field would be the psychiatrist's assertion that by charging the client high fees and ensuring that he pays them, the client will come to accept more responsibility for his treatment.

It is an interesting side light that in the late 70s when public funds for alcoholism treatment were relatively abundant, treatment personnel in Maine were very reluctant to impose fees on clients. They reasoned that to do so might deny service to clients "who really needed it", but could not afford it, or that if they could afford it, it tied the counselor up with paper work instead of the important issues of treatment, and finally that discussing such mundane issues as fees with clients might undermine the client/counselor relationship. Now that funds are growing scarcer, many programs are energetically pursuing fee collection, and the counselors are saying that fee payment is a sign of responsibility and recovery on the client's part and it is something counselors actively encourage as a therapeutic issue.

The ideology concerning the therapeutic impact of fee collection has changed dramatically. This change does not appear to have come about due to any controlled studies of the impact of fees on client outcome, but rather from the change in the importance of fees to the survival of the treatment organization.

This paper has described the adaptations of the staff of an alcoholism treatment program to the demands made on them in their environment. The adaptions took the form of an ideology emphasizing particular aspects of the clients or patients undergoing treatment in order to reduce the strains experienced by the staff. This form of adaptation is made possible by the fact that alcoholism treatment is not yet a well defined set of technical processes but rather a collection of ad hoc approaches each supported by a slightly different conceptual framework.

In recent years, the number and quality of evaluative studies of alcoholism treatment programs has greatly increased. It is possible that out of these studies a verifiable, and replicable treatment technology will emerge. As this technology emerges, the great debates that occur between the nationally recognized experts, and the small debates that occur between local treatment programs will be resolved. As treatment technology is refined and the debates subside, the opportunity of using a therapeutically based ideology to cope with role strains and problems will diminish. Since it is inevitable that such problems will continue to exist, treatment staffs will have to devise a new set of mechanisms to cope with them.

REFERENCES

Goode, W. J. A theory of role strains. *American Sociological Review,* 1960, 25, 483-496.

Malone, M., Berkowitz, N., & Klein, M. Interpersonal conflict in the out-patient department. *American Journal of Nursing,* 1962, 62, 108-118.

Moore, W. G. *The professions: Roles and rules.* New York: Russell Sage Foundation, 1970.

Parsons, T., & Fox, R. Illness, therapy and the modern family. In E. G. Jaco (Ed.), *A source book in behavioral science and medicine.* Glencoe, Ill.: Free Press, 1958.

Ryan, W. *Blaming the victim.* New York: Vintage (Random House), 1971.

Wechsler, H., & Rohman, M. Future caregiver's views on alcoholism treatment: A poor prognosis. *Journal of Studies on Alcohol,* 1982, 43, 939-955.

The Social Organization
of a Halfway House:
Relationship of a Dual Reality
Upon the Recovery
of Women Alcoholics

Joan N. Volpe, Ph.D.
James F. Rooney, Ph.D.

An important relationship exists between the organizational goals and program objectives of alcoholism treatment programs on the one hand, and the needs of clients in those programs on the other. This study investigates these relationships. It explores staff functioning, program objectives and client adaptations at a halfway house for recovering female alcoholics which we here call the Milestone.* The research is based on three years of field work in which participant observation was the primary research method used.

Because the halfway house contained either all or a large number of roles and activities of its residents, it had many of the characteristics of a "Total Institution" as described by Goffman (1961). Paramount among institutions of this sort are penitentiaries, asylums, military encampments, monasteries and convents. That the institutional setting contains all members' roles contrasts sharply to the usual situation in civil life where individuals tend to live in one place, work in another, and spend leisure time in still another. Also in civil life, there is not a unity of administrative control among these social spheres. Although the halfway house was not as self-contained as a penitentiary or an asylum, newcomers to the house did experience the life-style of a total institution until they found employment or in some other way extended their living space out-

Joan N. Volpe, Fairfax-Falls Church Community Services Board and James F. Rooney, Pennsylvania State University, Middletown, PA.

*A fictitious name given to the halfway house to protect the anonymity of the residents.

side the house. The degree to which the Milestone contained the roles of the residents varied with the resident's resources, such as possessing an automobile, employment, and outside friends. Those women who lacked these resources were totally dependent upon the house for food, shelter, recreation, and sociability.

Goffman describes the functioning of total institutions as marked almost universally by placing the needs and convenience of the staff and administrative ease over the needs of inmates. As is true of some self-serving bureaucracies, total institutions may not only place administrative convenience over client needs, but in many cases may actually subvert the organization's official purpose of rendering service or rehabilitation of inmates either because such subversion facilitates a less troubled operation for the staff or because it is necessary to insure the program's continued existence.

The issue of staff convenience and needs of clients is relevant in a variety of treatment settings besides total institutions. Bromet, et al. (1977) and Linn (1970) explored the relationship of staff expectations and client characteristics to treatment outcome. Ogborne's (1976) study of halfway houses suggests that it is the characteristics of the staff that determine their orientation toward clients rather than the objective characteristics or needs of the client population. If the social organization of halfway houses reflect staff needs or preferences at the expense of clients' needs, client progress may well be affected. In this chapter, we are interested in describing the Milestone's operative system in order to assess the degree to which the halfway house functioned to serve the recovery needs of the clients versus the need to perpetuate its own social organization.

RESEARCH PROCEDURES

In 1976, the female investigator made arrangements to visit a women's halfway house on a daily basis. These visits continued through February of 1979. The only restrictions placed on the investigator during the early phases of the project were to follow strict rules of confidentiality, to protect the women's anonymity at all times, and to remind residents that all conversations were completely voluntary.

Participant observation was the primary means of data collection. The value of this technique is that on-site observations allow the researcher to understand individuals or groups by becoming a part of their everyday reality. This form of data gathering elicits information about the fabric of life of a group which is rich and detailed far beyond what can be gathered by any sort of secondary source techniques such as test instruments and formal interviews.

Non-directed interviewing was the second most used data gathering technique. A non-scheduled interview guide (Richardson, 1965) was developed around specific classes of information that were of interest to the research team including client perceptions of the staff as role models; of the progress of their peers; and of the effectiveness of the halfway houses as a treatment setting in their own recovery.

For a six-month period in 1978, the time in which the Milestone had a structured treatment program, the investigator was a co-leader of group therapy at the Milestone. In addition to documenting the women's responses in this setting, each resident was asked to keep a notebook, or a diary, to record thought patterns, fears, feelings, needs, etc. Contents of these notebooks were shared with the investigator as yet another means to understand the phenomena of recovery. Data were continuously collected on the 71 women who resided at the halfway house over the three-year period. Special emphasis was placed on each resident's perceptions and behavior during the first 30 days, midway through the expected 90-day stay, and at discharge.

RESULTS

The major goal of the Milestone, like other halfway houses across the nation, is to provide direct assistance to alcoholics in the community. Structurally, these goals are met by offering residential shelter to alcoholic women, counseling to attain sobriety, transportation to Alcoholics Anonymous (AA) meetings, and support in the fellowship of AA. The cultural-institutional features of the halfway house are derived from the principles of Alcoholics Anonymous and from the experiences of sober alcoholics who reside in and visit the facility. According to halfway house policy, clients were expected to reside in the home for three months. The average length of stay, however, was 5.5 months.

For the majority of the clients residing in the halfway house during the three years of fieldwork, the Milestone house served, to a great extent, as an all-encompassing environment. Upon first entering the halfway house, nearly all women were both unemployed and penniless. Because they had no means to pay for outside entertainment, the unemployed residents of the Milestone of necessity spent nearly the entire day and night at the halfway house. For them, a day was passed by attending to chores and running a few necessary errands; all of which required no more than three hours. The remaining hours were usually spent at meals and in chatting and lounging around the house if there was not a therapy session being held.

For the most part, the Milestone house followed the organizational principles of halfway houses in this country; small size; simplicity of rules, reduction of status differences and informality (Rubington, 1967). However, in halfway houses, as in other organizations, the explicit or official goals may be opposed to underlying value patterns and, therefore, a system of conflicting goals or inconsistency may arise. This conflict was discovered in the halfway house social system through an analysis of the implicit rules as seen through the role performance of the individual participants.

Administratively, the halfway house had been staffed by recovered alcoholics who shared their own experiences of alcoholism with the residents and thereby set the official policy for alcoholism recovery. The staff and residents alike shared a distrust of "normies" (non-alcoholics) in the general population and also of "normie" professionals, in that the latter were believed to lack an understanding of the needs of the recovering alcoholic. With regard to treatment, the male administrative director of the halfway house believed that recovery was based on discipline, attendance at AA meetings and a sharing of alcoholic experiences. Organized treatment such as structured individual and group counseling, skills attainment, or employment training were out of his purview, and if desired, were to be acquired by the individual efforts of interested residents. This model of halfway house treatment was established years ago for the male clients of this treatment facility and was transferred without change to the newly opened women's component.

Conflict and imbalances in the organizational process of the halfway house were directly related to the divergence of power from the official channels to an unofficial or informal system. Lines of power became manifest in a double status system of "insiders" and "outsiders." As noted by Becker (1963), outsiders are individuals, who because of the possession of a critically disqualifying trait, or the performance of undesirable behavior, are considered morally inferior. Such persons are assumed to possess a very different motivation than members of the insider group, and for this reason, cannot be accepted into full community in that they cannot be trusted. Two bases of differentiation of insiders from outsiders were operative in the halfway house. One division of insiders versus outsiders recognized by house residents was based on alcoholic status. Among this group of recovering alcoholics, the world was divided into two categories of people: alcoholics and non-alcoholics. Anyone *not* an alcoholic was considered an outsider—a "normie," and was assumed not to understand how alcoholics really feel, think, and act. With the exception of one manager and her assistant, all staff and residents over the period of the study held insider status by being alcoholic as well as members of AA.

The most salient division of insiders from outsiders at the halfway house occurred in terms of allegiance or non-allegiance to the director and his interpretation of halfway house policy. Whether staff or resident, an "insider" was one who gave primary concern to organizational needs, i.e., to the policies, wishes, and whims of the director who held ultimate authority over the insider system. If, on the other hand, an individual's basic allegiance was tied to clients' concerns for recovery or treatment needs without regard for the director's policies, she was considered to be an outsider by the director's cadre who held power in the organization. Adhering to these implicit definitions as used at the Milestone, further references made to insider/outsider status in this chapter relate to organizational allegiances. The female cook, along with the assistant director and male cook at the men's houses held an insider's position in the organization in that they were dedicated to the director's policies regardless of the consequences for the welfare of individual residents. In varying degrees, all the managers held an outsider's status in the organization in that their primary allegiance was to better the condition of the clients. There was one exception. For a short period, a male manager assumed direction of the women's house. He was a loyal graduate of the men's halfway house as well as an active member of the board of directors and a firm believer in the director's policies.

The female cook had seniority at the halfway house and was commended for her loyalty and perseverance. Through times of hardship and joy she remained absolutely loyal to the director of the Milestone. Like mothers all over the world, this cook spent an inordinant amount of time fretting over her "children" while preparing and serving sumptuous meals. She soon became a matriarchal figure for residents, for managers, and most significantly for the director, who was served a special plate whenever he dined at the women's home.

The first three managers, although holding an insider status in AA, held an outsider's status in the organization. Each of their terms in office was marked by a series of attempts to gain insider status through being accepted by the power group which gave primary loyalty to the director. The attempt to gain insider status was accomplished by a variety of tactics, depending upon the personalities and needs of each individual. By the time the third manager was hired, the dual system was recognized by the residents themselves; there were actual discussions of factions or "camps" based on observations and judgments of the behavior of those who followed the organizational faction which was comprised of the director and his assistant, the male and the female cook, and those residents who gave allegiance to the director and his style of management.

Each of the women managers had varying degrees of conflict with the cook, and thereby with the director. Although there was little turmoil about treatment per se, since the early managers instituted few changes in the structure of the program, the female managers did believe that their women clients had special needs which differed from the male model of alcoholism treatment currently being used. Fear of change and non-compliance to the director's wishes sent the cook scurrying to the director with complaints regarding the management of the women's home. The consequence of the cook's actions was to neutralize the official flow of authority within the women's halfway house.

According to the dual reality based on the organization's power system, a "proper" resident was obliged to give ostensible behavioral and verbal support to both the formal and the informal systems of behavior in the house. But this meant that the outsiders were forced to make compromises if they wanted the shelter of this halfway house. The most flagrant compromise being asked of them related to their honesty. As recovering alcoholics they were learning through AA that honesty with self and others was essential to sobriety. However, if they followed the teachings of AA to communicate their feelings openly, they were thwarted by the official system of the Milestone which demanded that one cover up infractions of staff members and some residents. According to reports from staff and residents, these infractions included such activities as taking large quantities of food from the kitchen for personal use, dipping into petty cash, and inefficient management of the prescription medicine. If for instance, a resident delayed completing an assigned chore by the appointed hour, the manager might decide that an individual counseling session was more appropriate than completing the task. This practice soon infuriated the cook who believed that clients were manipulating management in order to avoid their assigned work. While this may have been partially true, the cook was very agitated over individual counseling sessions because they were a form of information control (confidentiality) which threatened her power. The director taking a non-directive approach, wanted to avoid conflict when informed of happenings at the women's home. Therefore, when personalities clashed or treatment policies were in dispute, he relinquished his authoritative role and assumed a position of quiet indifference. When the conflict continued beyond his level of patience, the female manager was asked to leave her position.

At that point in the history of the corporation, the Board of Directors became concerned over the high turnover of personnel and there was some discussion that possibly the manager of the women's home should be directly responsible to the board of directors, and thereby out of the line of management of the director. However, this change never materialized. To smooth ruffled feathers, the director asked a male graduate of his program, formerly trained as a psychologist to manage the women's home. During this period, the director received few complaints from the cook about the management of the women's home. However, the clients were bored and restless. The halfway house offered no treatment, but served instead as a shelter for the women residents. Because the male manager was a product of the men's home and had a long allegiance to the director, the dialogue regarding separate factions dissipated. During this period, all halfway house staff were insiders in terms of allegiance to the organization and residents were either insiders or recalcitrant alcoholics.

Insiders of the organization were bound together through reciprocity in the bestowal of special favors. This held true for staff and residents alike. For example, if the female cook chose to spend the evening away from the halfway house on a night when she was officially listed as the employee on duty, insider residents would cover by assuming such routine activities as answering phones, checking on resident curfews, and locking the doors in the evening. These insider residents also held the phone number where the cook could be reached in case an emergency arose and the cook needed to return quickly to the halfway house. Information about the cook's evasion of responsibility rarely reached the director, partly because of an allegiance to the cook which was rewarded by favors, and partly because the residents wished to avoid additional conflict. In return for this allegiance, insider residents were not reprimanded if they broke a curfew, were lax in their household duties, or started gossip in the house.

Outsiders were rarely confronted by insiders when conflict arose. Rather, the cook would gather her cadre of insider residents at the breakfast table (usually before the managers came on duty in the morning) to "discuss" the behavior of a particular resident. Of course, the individual in question would hear about all the comments which were made. If the client lost her temper to the cook or another insider, the client was labeled a troublemaker. If, on the other hand, the accused calmly discussed the problem with the cook, more often than not there was a denial by the cook that any such statement was made. And so the system of backbiting and deception continued until the outsider left the halfway house. If the resident left sober, there was continous talk concerning how long she would "make it" with her attitude. If she was discharged for drinking, the cook and other insiders would remark, "Well, I told you she wasn't serious about her sobriety." In these cases, the cook's evaluation of a client's recovery program was positively reinforced by insider residents and the director: "Leave it to the cook; she can really spot the serious clients from the hangers-on." The female managers recognized the dynamics of the vindictive system, but were powerless to change it.

Outsider residents were outraged by the organizational inconsistencies and the favoritism. Their anger, sometimes out of proportion to the importance of the incident, led to internal fighting and open hostility. For the insiders, the behavior of the outsiders was explained as an indication that these women were not ready to give up their alcoholic ways, i.e., they were belligerent, manipulative, secretive troublemakers. According to one outsider resident: "If you don't walk the walk and talk the talk of the Milestone, you cannot make it in this system."

There was one case of an outsider resident who had had an experience in group living in a religious order before coming to the house. Out of her personal experience of communal systems, she believed that for self-preservation it was necessary to fight a system which allowed flagrant abuse of house rules. She maintained her integrity by eliciting support from other outsider residents while continuing to live up to her responsibility as a house member. Although there had been previous residents who had attempted to stand up to the system, all others had chosen for personal reasons to leave the organization and continue recovery elsewhere. This particular resident, however, felt a personal obligation to remain in the house. During her stay, the' workings of the dual system reached a high level of turmoil, especially when she and other outsider residents spoke at a house AA meeting about the discrepancies between the AA program and the house system. Although temporary minor changes were made to placate these residents, the inner conflict continued. When this resident chose to leave, the cook and other insiders branded her as an ungrateful, destructive busybody. But the cook's power extended beyond the formal roles of the women's house. While it was a common practice that all former residents were encouraged to return to the Milestone for a weekly AA meeting, the cook was able to manipulate the formal system and have this privilege rescinded for the "troublemaking" resident. A few days after discharge, the resident who fought the system received a letter from the secretary to the director informing her that she was no longer welcome at the halfway house, nor was she to transport former residents to AA meetings at the house.

The above incident occurred during the period when the house was managed by two non-alcoholic women: a manager and assistant manager. The assistant manager was placed in the house under the Comprehensive Employment Training Act (CETA). These women were hired after the male manager retired. The administrative director would have preferred hiring alcoholic women, but there were no eligible candidates for the position.

This period in the history of the house was marked by external changes in local mental health agency policy and a demand for strict record keeping for the use of all Federal Title XX funds (the source of monies allocated to assist alcoholics in recovery). The non-alcoholic managers brought professionalism to the halfway house. Client forms were efficiently and systematically filed. A treatment program was designed and utilized. The selection process of incoming residents was tightened.

These managers, like the other women managers in the past, were told by the director that the women's home was in their charge as long as the written rules of abstinence and curfew were complied with. However, little training was given to the non-alcoholic managers and even less guidance regarding administrative policies was offered concerning the decision making process. These managers having a total outsider status, i.e., not members of AA and not having allegiance to the organizational system, approached their duties believing they had the power to manage. However, they soon found that if their decisions contradicted the latent system of the organization, covert conflict arose. Through a grapevine of outsider residents, the new managers learned when insiders (management and residents) were displeased with their work. Occasionally, the female managers would confront the director asking for clarification or guidance. With the exception of open discussion of a few specific mundane problems, the issue of discomfort was specifically avoided in staff discussion.

The major issue of conflict was the existence of a treatment program and the non-alcoholic status of the managers. Although the director had approved the treatment program design, the cook and the most senior residents, who had been part of the system prior to the term of present management, firmly believe that non-alcoholics could not assist alcoholics and, therefore, felt that group therapy should not be obligatory for them. Their position was sustained by the director. As a result, the insider/outsider delineations became more complex. Additional boundaries were added which served to delineate those residents who believed non-alcoholics could counsel alcoholics and those who maintained that only an alcoholic can understand another alcoholic.

Conflict continued and expanded. Bonds of affiliation grew and were more clearly demarcated. The staff became the butt of the morning gossip-mongering. Those residents who believed they were being helped by the staff were in a terrible quandary trying to deal with in-group feelings between alcoholics in AA meetings and out-group feelings towards those alcoholics in the house who were part of the Milestone system and, therefore, opposed to professionalism.

Although incoming residents received the benefits of the new treatment program, confusion reigned in the house. Open communication which existed in group therapy could not be transferred out of the group. New skills for living could only be utilized when they did not conflict with the cook's idea of rehabilitation for alcoholics. One of the residents summed up her feelings regarding the conflict in management after she had been reprimanded by the cook for not attending to her duties. Addressing the cook, she said:

"You're crazy—you walk around here picking on everyone. Your tongue is the devil's workshop. You cause more people to go back to drinking with your tongue. It's more dangerous than a sword." At this point, the cook turned to the resident saying: "Pack your bags. I have the authority to kick you out. So get out." The resident went to the telephone and reported the incident to a relative by saying: "I've been thrown out of here for not vacuuming before noon—a rule which was never explained to me. This is supposed to be a loving place which cares for sick people, but I'm thrown out for not vacuuming on time."

Many of the new residents turned to the managers to relieve the organizational pressure. But the managers were unable to eliminate the conflict because they had no power either to restrain or fire the cook. The organizational chart of halfway house authority was skewed since the cook had a direct line of communication with the director, who took a non-direct approach. In his words, "All I want is peace in that women's home, and all I have is trouble. When will I find a woman who knows how to run that place? I don't have time to run the women's and the men's homes, too!"

In time, the complaints from the cook and insider resdents grew to such proportions that the director suggested to the women managers that they reduce the amount of therapy given, counsel only on demand, and stop using a psychological approach with the clients. Although the managers did not give up (or give in), their enthusiasm waned. The treatment program became more unstructured and basically was at the discretion of the client. If a client wanted counseling, she would receive it; if she chose not to participate, she was allowed to use the house as a shelter.

Seven months after joining the staff, the manager heard from the cook at the men's house that she was going to be fired and that the director wanted to hire an alcoholic manager. In order to avoid being discharged from her position, she gave notice and left the halfway house. The assistant manager, under contract to the Comprehensive Employment Training Act, had two more months on the job. She was allowed to finish out her term of work. In a few weeks a recovered female alcoholic who was a registered nurse, filled the manager's position. One of the first decisions the new manager made was to curtail the activities of the cook. With the concurrence of the director, it was agreed that the cook would be closely monitored and held strictly accountable for her hours on duty and for the use of petty cash. Although there was never a problem regarding the cook being available for duties during the daytime, the manager would personally check to see that she was actually on the premises during the nights that she was the official employee on duty. All expenditures out of petty cash were to be strictly accounted for by itemized receipts. Furthermore, the morning informal "counseling" sessions in the dining room were to be ended; the cook was not to volunteer her advice on any matter other than the management of the kitchen. Although the cook resented these restrictions, this manager was able to curtail her longstanding activities.

Although successful, the restrictions this manager placed on the cook did not last long. After three weeks the cook and two insider residents went to the director and testified that the manager had been seen drinking. This placed the director in a "no-win situation" in that he suspected the motives of the cook, yet he felt he could not afford to keep anyone on the staff who would ever be suspected of having taken a drink. Choosing the safer course of insuring that the reputation of "his staff" was above reproach, the director asked the manager to leave her post for allegedly breaking the abstinence rule.

The women's house then came under new management for the seventh time during the three years of field work. The next manager was a recovering female alcoholic who believed that non-alcoholic professionals have a place in the world of alcoholic services. This belief was not consonant with that of the director and directly conflicted with that of the cook. Initially the new manager made no changes in program or policy. She did, however, keep careful detailed notes on the cook's behavior. After three weeks and while still on her probationary period, she approached the director of the corporation and confronted him with documentation of the cook's behavior. She informed the director that she did not want to put the cook out in the street, since the Milestone had become her home. Instead, the manager insisted that the cook would either have to comply with her rules as manager or once again would either become a resident in treatment. The director agreed with the manager's suggestions including one that the cook take a forced two week vacation.

When she first returned from the vacation, the cook's behavior was more subdued. Within a few weeks, however, she slowly started to build her power base to once again become a covert leader by offering extra food to certain residents. The manager warned the cook about her transgressions and informed the director concerning the problem situation. At this point an important unplanned event occurred; one of the two women's houses had a fire and it was necessary to move all women into the larger's women's house. Because of the overcrowding in the one remaining women's facility and because there was extra space in one of the men's houses, the cook's living quarters were moved to a nearby men's house. That men's house served as the central kitchen and dining room for both houses. In the new setting the cook had no one to counsel, no recipient of her favors and no way to rebuild a following. Although the women came to the men's house, each remained only long enough to eat. The men did not become suitable clients for building a covert group of insiders. The cook's functions quickly became limited solely to cooking. Approximately four months after the fire, she suffered a nervous breakdown and eventually was asked to leave the Milestone.

IMPLICATIONS FOR TREATMENT

The dual system of social reality described above operated within the halfway house over the three years of fieldwork. What was the effect of this dual reality upon the recovery process of women residents? Although idiosyncratic reactions to the Milestone's social organization did emerge, various patterns of responses also became evident. A useful perspective for studying responses of residents to an institutionalized setting is provided by Erving Goffman (1961). Goffman's analytic scheme of institutionalized adaptations has been applied to this halfway house study as a means of understanding the various reactions adopted by the women residents to manage the social reality of the Milestone. Of particular importance is the relationship between the various adaptations and the women's recovery at the Milestone.

In his analysis of total institutions, Goffman (1961) lists five major modes of adaptation made by residents to the lifeway of institutional settings: situational withdrawal, intransigency, colonization, conversion, and playing it cool. This classification constituted a repertoire of responses, and any particular individual may practice any one or a combination of these behaviors at various times and in various circumstances throughout the stay in the institution. Each of the adaptive behaviors occurred at the Milestone.

Situational withdrawal involves withdrawing apparent attention from all situations and persons except the most immediately surrounding events. This occurred among Milestone residents most frequently during their first month of residence. Although psychological withdrawal was influenced by the process of physiological recovery from acute drinking states, we believe of more importance is the emotional devastation which occurs through the recognition of having lost a major part of one's denial system regarding the seriousness of one's drinking. The fact that a woman has come to have no other alternative but to enter a rehabilitation facility for alcoholics constitutes an undeniable manifestation of a severe alcohol problem. The occurrence of situational withdrawal varied principally according to whether or not a client had been in another treatment facility immediately before entering the Milestone. Severe withdrawal occurred more frequently among women who entered the house without having been in any prior treatment or who came from a seven-day detoxification center in that they had less time to recognize and to accept their alcoholic status than those entering from a 28-day treatment center.

Goffman's second adaptation, the *intransigent line,* consists of open, intentional refusal to cooperate with the staff. Although there were many times when various members failed to perform their assigned house duties and at other times were in some ways defiant of managerial authority, consistent and open intransigency seldom occurred. Its relative absence is due principally to the fact that, in contrast to prisons and for many patients in asylums, entrance is legally voluntary and continued residence is at the pleasure of the administration. Because residence at the facility was seen to be contingent upon continued good behavior, those women who wanted an excuse to leave the house and go out and drink again could find it through defiant refusal to perform expected duties. Such persons ostensibly were asked to leave the Milestone because they had "poor attitude." Having left under these conditions, a woman felt very justified in returning to drinking as proper compensation for her deprivations.

Another adaptation, *colonization,* is the construction of a relatively stable, contented existence out of the resources and satisfactions available within the institution. Once constructed, the constellation of assets is viewed as in many ways superior to life on the outside. Colonization or the building of an advantageous niche in the Milestone social system occurred principally by forming a sexual liaison with an insider resident of the men's houses. Thereafter the woman would be treated as an insider in the organization. The man chosen must be an insider in one of the men's houses, a person who affirmed the organization's ways. A relationship either with a male outsider resident or with some other members of Alcoholics Anonymous was a means of receiving better treatment in the women's house. When a liaison was formed, it was very much like the institution of "going steady" in high school, the particular woman became "spoken for," and was socially restricted and sexually not approachable by other men in the Milestone. Critical to this alliance, her status in the women's house changed through a communication from the cook at the men's house, informing the female cook of the existence of the personal relationship; and that thereafter, the woman was not to be hassled.

Conversion occurs when a client or inmate takes on the official staff view as a self-image and tries to act out the role of the perfect group member. The circle of organizational insiders in the Milestone consists of those who hold personal allegiance to the director and his interpretation of the proper method of rehabilitation of alcoholics, regardless of its degree of suitability for particular residents. The insiders thus did not develop personal or organizational links outside the halfway house, but rather restricted their purview to the Milestone corporation, which for them was very much a total institution. Like converts in many other types of total institutions, the insiders felt a great degree of security and reinforcement through their identification with the policies and practices of the officially appointed management.

Playing it cool is defined by Goffman as the opportunistic combination of secondary adjustments, colonization, conversion, yet ostensible manifestation of loyalty to the official culture so as to maximize the chance of getting out psychologically undamaged. To Goffman's criteria, we might add that playing it cool is practiced for the objective reason of seeking to minimize the chance of trouble with either the staff or with other inmates. Goffman notes that this is the adaptation followed by the greatest number of residents in total institutions. Playing it cool in the Milestone was accomplished by giving a public verbal commitment to the wishes of the cook and the director, while maintaining a private level of personal integrity which left the individual some degree of choice in her rehabilitative efforts. Because one's actions were not determined, residents referred to this system of behavior as a survival technique in which they "talked the talk, but don't have to walk the walk." These residents, for example, would sit quietly at the dining room table during discussion of the cook's abuse of rules and privileges, but they would only minimally join the gossip. On the other hand, they would refuse to become recipients of special favors proffered by the cook. Women who chose this strategy seemed to have a quasi-insider/-outsider position since neither of the groups could assess the women's motives. If their personalities were winsome, they were to find a niche in the system.

The previous section reveals the existence of a privileged system and adaptive alignment in the halfway house which parallel those of total institutions. However, unlike total institutions which possess a monolithic reality, the halfway house for alcoholics functions in terms of two major principles: (1) an ideology found on the principles of Alcoholics Anonymous (a cultural reality) and (2) the formal organizational system of the halfway house (the institutional reality). When these two systems were incongruent, individuals residing in the halfway house face life with a series of contradictions.

A sober way of life advanced in AA speaks of honesty to self and to others, reduction of manipulation, alleviation of resentments, open communication, identification of feelings, and constructive action. Residents come to the halfway house to learn these skills and understandably they turn to the halfway house staff as role models in the assimilation of this new way of life.

In the early stages of recovery, muddle-headedness caused by alcoholism keeps the residents in a state of confusion. Few personal or social alignments were made until the women felt they were somewhat capable of assessing the situation. Those residents who had lived in other institutions were cautious, leery, and somewhat aware of modes of adaptation to an institution. But for those women who had no previous institutional experience, life in the halfway house was especially devastating in that they lacked the necessary skills of adaptation, particularly of playing it cool by giving verbal assent to the house policies while utilizing the program to seek their private objectives. Those who became insiders gave their primary allegiance to the organizational system. When there was conflict between principles of AA and the operating procedures of the organization, insiders consistently supported the organization's position. The other women, however, whose primary allegiance was to Alcoholics Anonymous, had a problematic existence in the halfway house, since they were outsiders from the organizational system. Outsider residents, then, were those women who developed and maintained relationships with members of AA and/or individual friends. Due in part to the assistance of the outsider social support, these women found that they could maintain a level of personal integrity and remain at the house while they recovered. To exist within the institutional system, however, they had to con, manipulate, and hide many of their fears and feelings. For many of the residents this dual system of realities was especially devastating. Their feelings of frustration, powerlessness and hopelessness grew until they could take some form of affirmative action. As one resident said after attending an institutional banquet:

> My anger at the house program was so strong as I sat and listened to the speakers at the banquet talk about their indebtedness to the Milestone. How can they be so dishonest, so hypocritical? At the women's home, you can't use your integrity and have a freedom of choice. I don't want to play their games, but I have to survive. I have no other place to live. All I do is internalize this anger and I know how self-destructive that is. But tonight I lost it, sitting there listening to people praise a system that is sick, sicker than we are. I just felt as if there is no way to win, and before I knew it, I was having a compulsive reaction to drink. That is why I must be honest with feelings. I don't want to drink, and I feel I am sinking.

Some residents succumbed to those feelings of helplessness and suffered a relapse into drinking. Others, like the women quoted above, chose to live a dual reality, using conning strategies of survival to exist within the system, and open communication with folks outside the institution. For women in a recovery situation, living a dual life was a tremendous emotional burden taking a great deal of self-discipline and a strong commitment to sobriety.

Conflict between organizational needs, as seen in staff behavior and program objectives were observed during the three years of field work in this halfway house for alcoholic women. Throughout the data gathering period, the authors wondered how the halfway house conflict might be affecting the recovery of the residents. Without a comparison group of alcoholic women, it was not possible to discern, with any degree of confidence, the relationship between staff functioning and client progress. However, a system's approach to human behavior would clearly point to the connectedness of staff functioning, role modeling, and client adaptations.

Participant observation indicated that halfway houses, as treatment settings, have some characteristics of the "total institution."

In fact, the women residents in this house manifested some of the same adaptations documented by Goffman's work in the mental institution (1961). With regard to specific adaptations and alcohol recovery, one might speculate that the adaptation of *playing it cool* might have had little adverse effect upon a resident's recovery, but that *conversion* could be particularly damaging for the woman alcoholic whose sobriety necessitates the development of independence and autonomy.

Results of this research indicate that there is a relationship between official goals, informal organizational structure, and treatment outcome. From the data gathered in this exploratory study, the authors hypothesize that when organizational goals conflict with program objectives, clients assume survival adaptations that contraindicate long-term sobriety. While informal follow-up of the women residents in this halfway house appears to support this hypothesis, a rigorous study design is needed to validate the effects of organizational conflict and long-term sobriety.

REFERENCES

Becker, H. S. *Outsiders: Studies in the Sociology of Deviance.* New York: The Free Press. 1963.

Bromet, E., Moos, R.; Wuthmann, C. and Bliss, F. Treatment experiences of alcoholic patients; an analysis of five residential alcoholism programs. *International Journal of the Addictions* 12:953-958. 1977.

Goffman, E. *Asylums.* Garden City: Doubleday and Co. 1961.

Linn, L. S. State hospital environment and rates of patient discharge. *Archives Of General Psychiatry* 23:346-351. 1970.

Ogborne, A. C. and Smart, R. G. Halfway houses for skid row alcoholics; are they rehabilitative? *Addictive Behaviors* 1:305-309. 1976.

Richardson, S., Dohrenwend, B., and Klein, D. *Interviewing—Its Forms and Functions,* New York: Basic, 1965.

Rubington, E. The halfway house for the alcoholic. *Mental Hygiene* 51:552-560. 1967.

Gender-Role Dynamics
in an Alcohol Therapy Group

S. Priyadarsini

INTRODUCTION

In our society, traditionally women are considered expressive, integrative in their orientations while men are defined as instrumental beings (Duberman, 1977). That is, women engage in tension management, emotional nurturance, support, and affection and men are the major decision-makers and problem-solvers. The cultural stereotype of the sexes is an extension of these definitions; women are portrayed as passive, weak, unthinking, emotional, intuitive, self-sacrificing, practical, narcissistic, dependent, inconsistent, and helpless while men are pictured as being strong, dependable, unemotional, rational, coherent, brave, and intelligent (Duberman, 1977). Thus, there is a cultural notion that men and women are different. Hence, it is not surprising that, from time to time, writers in the field of alcohol studies have raised the issue of the distinction between male and female alcoholics.

Early on, researchers (Lisansky, 1957) in the field have recognized the lack of, and need for, empirical research on women alcoholics. Curlee (1967), for example, criticized the prevalent studies as either ignoring women entirely or assuming that alcoholism is the same for both sexes. Since then, research and literature in the field have come to describe, compare, and contrast male and female alcoholics' demographic and personality profiles, behavior, and prognosis. Several studies demonstrate the gender-based differences among alcoholics. For example, hospitalized alcoholic men, compared with their female counterparts, claim to have consumed more alcohol, had more arrests, and lost more jobs and friends because of their drinking (Rimmer et al., 1971). Curlee (1970) reported that more of the women than men alcoholics were divorced, admitted as

The author would like to thank the Center of Alcohol Studies, Rutgers University and Clayton A. Hartjen, Jayshree Parthasarathy, and Lucile Duberman.

psychiatric patients, admitted more often, and for longer periods of time. Female alcoholics are said to differ from male alcoholics in yet other ways: women alcoholics tend to exhibit greater variability and pathological gender-role orientations, sexual promiscuity, disruptions of social ties, physiological precipitants of drinking (Lisansky, 1957; Kinsey, 1966; Wilsnack, 1973, 1976; Saunders, 1980). Women, more than men, alcoholics admit to broken marriages and having attempted suicide (Rothod and Thomson, 1971). Female alcoholics, in contrast to males, tend to perceive themselves as having psychiatric problems (Tamerin, 1978).

It has been found that unlike men who engage in convivial drinking, women alcoholics tend to engage in solitary drinking (Pemberton, 1967). According to several writers, women alcoholics are more subject to social sanctions and stigma than are alcoholic men (Lisansky, 1957, 1958; Curlee, 1968, 1970; Schmidt and de Lint, 1969; Rothod and Thomson, 1971; Wilsnack, 1973). Women alcoholics reportedly have poorer prognosis than alcoholic men (Bateman and Petersen, 1972; Schuckit and Morissey, 1976). Women alcoholics seem to prefer individual therapy, while alcoholic men show a preference for group therapy (Curlee, 1971). In short, there are a number of important differences between female and male alcoholics.

Do the differences between male and female alcoholics have implications for treatment strategies and outcomes? A few studies refer to various issues concerning the assumptions underlying the standard treatment strategies, most of which are based on experiences with male alcoholics or in coed sessions (Schuckit and Morissey, 1976). The need for different approaches to the treatment of male and female alcoholics has also been emphasized by some authors (Beckman, 1975; Greenblatt and Schuckit, 1976; Tamerin et al., 1976). Wilsnack (1976) remarks that the major fallacy when the same treatment is rendered to both gender groups is the assumption that both sexes drink excessively for the same reason. She points out, for example, that alcoholic women place great importance on their traditional, familial roles. Thus, it is likely that gender-related similarities and dissimilarities would have some importance for treatment strategies and, therefore, prognosis.

Observations conducted by the author of single-sex and coed group treatment sessions over several weeks suggest that not only do men and women alcoholics behave differently in group sessions, but each group focuses on different yet specific aspects of their day-today roles. These observations were conducted over a five-week period in a private, residential therapeutic community in the northeastern United States. All persons observed knew that the researcher was "observing," but were not aware of the purpose of the observations. Since no explicit hypotheses guided the research, the observations were unstructured. Field notes were completed daily to avoid any errors from introspective recollection. The facility was observed from 8:30 a.m. to 4:00 p.m. every weekday, plus a few weekend sessions. Since two group sessions were in progress simultaneously, an attempt was made to cover an equal number of sessions led by each of the counselors.

THE TREATMENT FACILITY AND ITS RESIDENTS

The facility is located on the outskirts of a historic town in an old, small, hospital building. It has ties to a major hospital which served at times as the conduit for recruiting residents, whom the staff referred to as "patients." Both the staff and patients treated the facility as if it were a medical unit. At any time there were about 30 patients in residence. They generally claimed to have come for treatment voluntarily, although the staff stated that there were pressures such as the employer's or spouse's ultimatum that the patient receive treatment.

Upon arrival, whether from a detoxification unit or otherwise, the patients were isolated from the outside world and made to immerse totally in themselves and the life of the therapeutic community. This suspension of contact with family and friends continued for a week or so. Patients spent a minimum of four weeks in treatment. Although there were a few patients who came in for counseling, the observations reported here are based on the "inpatient" segment of the patient population.

The patients seemed to be middleclass males and females. The male patients' occupations covered the spectrum of middleclass pursuits—from writer to heavy, construction equipment mover. All seemed to have completed at least high school, and, all except one, were currently employed. A majority of the women were not employed and a few were in white-collar jobs; they seemed to be the wives, mothers, or daughters of men who were engaged in various middleclass occupations. All of the patients paid for their treatment directly out of their pockets, or indirectly via their insurance companies; none were on medicare or medicaid.

The staff consisted of eight counselors, two physicians, several nursing, clerical, and other support personnel. Five of the counselors were nonalcoholics while the other three were "recovering" alcoholics who were active participants in Alcoholics Anonymous (AA). The latter were about fifty plus years of age while the others were younger (late 20's and 30's). Three of the counselors were female. Although on occasional days female residents outnumbered the males, typically about half of the patients were women. The women occupied adjacent (shared) rooms along one side of the corridor, while the men were in the other wing of the corridor.

The official day in the facility began at 8:30 a.m. with a staff meeting that usually lasted for 30 minutes. Then, at 10:00 a.m., the first two group sessions led by the counselors began. The afternoons began with a coed "lecture" at 1:00 p.m. that lasted for about an hour. "Lectures" consisted of listening to an AA volunteer; sometimes, professionals such as dieticians delivered informative lectures; or, an AA tape was played in the presence and leadership of an AA volunteer. Lectures were followed by a 30 minute "walking" period for those residents permitted to engage in such physical activities. At 2:30 p.m., two other group therapy sessions under the guidance counselors began and lasted for about 90 minutes. The evenings and weekends consisted of more such scheduled activities.

FINDINGS

One specific aspect—the gender component—of the interaction among the participants in the group sessions is the focus of this paper. The quality of the sessions varied somewhat depending upon the personality, background, and other idiosyncracies of the individual counselors. However, depending upon the gender of the patients, certain patterns in the following aspects of the groups' dynamics were observable: (1) initiative taken in introducing topics for discussion, (2) the topics and issues discussed, (3) formality of demeanor and language, and (4) level of affectivity exhibited.

Initiative

Most of the male residents took greater initiative in starting the group sessions. They were also less resistant to discussing any topic. Even the taboo subject of sex was raised by one patient who wanted the symbolism and meanings of his sex-related nightmares discussed in the group. Even the less articulate of the males brought up issues and topics they wanted discussed in group, and only a few had to be specifically addressed before they would speak.

On the other hand, in the female group sessions, unless specifically called upon, most did not initiate discussions. There were quite a few who did not say much even when prompted. When counselors addressed specific females by asking "How are you?," the typical response tended to be "OK!" followed by dead silence. Two specific incidents may suggest why this was the case.

When a counselor asked how everyone was doing, the women in unison responded "fine!". Immediately they all broke into a nervous laughter and someone remarked that they were doing the same thing that they did when their alcoholism set in—that is, say things were fine when they were not. One patient, who seemed quite concerned about speaking her mind for fear of being "analyzed," remarked that if she said anything other than "fine," she felt funny and embarrassed, since if she said that something was wrong, her motives become circumspect. In fact, she was pointing out a basic contradiction between AA ideology that emphasizes honesty, and the tendency of the treatment personnel to attribute negative meaning to some patients' honesty. The staff seemed to think that this patient demanded a lot of attention and felt threatened if anyone else got any attention from her fellow patients or the staff. It is hard to say to what extent the silence of these women indicates negative social emotional behavior due to either passive rejection or withdrawal out of the group (see Bales, 1950). A similar tendency to keep things private was indicated in yet another patient's complaint against a counselor who asked her to discuss a letter she was proposing to write to her daughter. The patient claimed it was a personal business between her and her child.

The seeming lack of initiative on the part of the women became even more noticeable in the coed sessions when even the few talkative females "clammed up." In contrast to the women, some of the male residents blatantly mentioned that since they were paying for it one way or another, they were going to get as much as they could out of the program by asking questions and raising issues that were bothering them.

Topics Discussed

Whether the group leader was male or female, the male residents typically raised, discussed, and focused on work-related problems.

These varied among topics such as the nature and worthwhileness of their jobs, drinking on the job, the frustrations and aggravations of work, relations with one's coworkers and boss, the questions and attitudes of those in the work place when one returns to work, and finding and changing jobs. Even the younger men talked about their future strictly in terms of their jobs. One male patient, for instance, was warned by the group not to slip if he doesn't find a job soon after he "graduated"; he was advised to "hang in there." Looking introspective, another man narrated his frustrations when he was once asked to dismantle a sales operation he had built up. Another expressed resentment that his boss sometimes asked him to do something that he felt was beneath his rank and experience. A third patient discussed his conflict with his coworker in his maintenance job. A younger patient lamented his demotion from his waiter's job and mentioned how ashamed he was of the fact that all the "girls" hired along with him were moving up.

Another work-role related preoccupation of the males surfaced on several different occasions. Some of the men apparently envied the sophistication and articulateness of those peers in treatment whom they defined as "successful" and openly admitted their feelings of inferiority in terms of their occupation and training. One patient, a writer, was the particular object of resentment by some of the other men. One referred to him as a creative person; a second called him a thinker and a smart person; and a third stated that he was envious of the writer's way with words. And the object of envy was warned by the group not to "intellectualize" too much. One patient occasionally went into a tirade indicating his preoccupation with success and prestige. He sarcastically remarked how the successful, snooty guys in their three-piece suits and fancy "air-conditioned" cars wouldn't bother rolling down their windows to hand the plastic (credit) card to him when he was working in a gas station. On another occasion, one man remarked that it is strange how the three martinis drunk by executives at lunch time seemed okay, but a beer-drinking working man is branded an alcoholic. Another talked about his wife being more educated and having a more prestigious job than he, admitting that he had an "inferiority complex" about it all. This man also defined as successful a person who has three cars when he himself had only one.

A third aspect of work that was the focus of concern centered upon its effects on sobriety. For example, one resident was asked by his peers if his job was worth "all the frustrations taken out on beer.'' Concern was expressed about a resident returning to the same job that seemed to have created his frustrations in the first place. Other common topics concerned matters such as being over-qualified, lack of job definition, and having too many bosses to answer to.

Thus, for the men, work was a prime concern. The women, on the other hand, exhibited less of a preoccupation with such work relationships. Only two mentioned their work since they were the only ones to have been employed at the time of treatment. One, for instance, described how her self-administered valium withdrawal (on the advice of her physician) made her dysfunctional at work; she connected the wrong persons when several phones started ringing simultaneously. The other employed woman was more concerned about her hatred for one ''nosy'' coworker who would be curious to know where she had been while absent from work.

In contrast to men, the women were more preoccupied with their social network—their traditional, expressive and affective role orientations to those around them. For example, one patient mentioned how when her husband was making only $5 per week, she was making twice that much, although she wouldn't dare remind him of that except when he was in a ''good mood.'' One day, a woman patient complained about the disappearance of a $20 bill from her billfold. The women were unhappy at the innuendo but still wouldn't offend the other woman. None of them said anything, although there was tension. In the end, one gathered enough courage to point out that it was impossible that it would be missing from her billfold since all their money was impounded and locked away upon their arrival at the facility. One woman complained that she could never say ''no'' when neighbors and acquaintances roped her into various voluntary work such as baking for a cake sale.

In addition, the major focus of their discussion was with expressing their honest feelings and emotions—letting their hair down. They talked at great length about being ''people pleaser'' (as one woman familiar with AA argot put it). They claimed they could never articulate their anger, resentments or anything that might sound negative or displeasing (Blume, 1978).

One woman complained at length about her sister-in-law's attempts to dictate her vacation plans. Another discussed her fury when her sister-in-law gave her crystals knowing fully well that the former had a drinking problem. This patient narrated another vignette—her mother-in-law had the habit of buying her curtains unasked; but this patient dare not tell her mother-in-law that she would rather choose her own. Another woman was in tears out of fear that her brother and one son were colluding to sell and displace her from the family home to which she was very attached. She felt unable to communicate her feelings and persuade them not to sell the house. However, the women, unlike the men, tended to breakdown and cry a lot. One broke out in tears upon learning that the staff recommended an extension of her stay. Whether this can be interpreted as expressing one's feelings honestly cannot be asserted. Although she would not divulge her reasons in the group, she later confided to the researcher that she was worried about her ability to pay for it.

One woman remarked that her mother somehow manages to make her feel guilty for not being the same as she was—happy, spontaneous, gregarious, and "full of life." While these women focused a great deal of attention on such expressive-affective components of their traditional roles, the men talked about the destructive ways in which they expressed their feelings of anger; or, as one put it, the "inappropriate" ways in which they took out their frustrations.

Unlike the men, the women patients were concerned with explaining to their friends, neighbors, and acquaintances their absence while in treatment. They were eager to discuss the details of how, and to whom to explain their absence, treatment, and alcoholism. An entire session was spent in role-playing for such contingencies.

The women conveyed the importance of their traditional roles in several references to the pressures of trying to be "supermoms" (Kinsey, 1966; Lisansky, 1957; Pemberton, 1967). Only one man ever mentioned his domestic role related frustrations. He hated painting his house but did it anyhow because, as he put it, "someone had to do it." This, like the general inattention to interpersonal matters paid by the men, was said in passing and more as an introspective remark than as a "complaint." Similarly, one man briefly mentioned how his children were "all grown up" before he realized that he hadn't spent any time playing and doing things with them. Another claimed that he still doesn't understand his children's ways, although "I am no Archie Bunker." Yet another expressed concern with his six-year old's well-being if he were to leave his alcoholic wife in order to maintain his sobriety. Another claimed that he was the buffer between his old-fashioned well-to-do parents and rebellious older siblings. One man gleefully narrated an incident involving his (now ex-) wife's embarrassment when his dog urinated on the fender of his sportscar she and her lover were driving. Another indicated that he did not realize the extent of his family's concern about his drinking. One of the patients mentioned how one could not patch up a broken marriage and another expressed fear of losing his wife because her parents were against him. In brief, although concern regarding interpersonal relationships surfaced in the men's sessions, it was not the main focus of attention nor did the men dwell on the topic.

Formality of Demeanor and Language

Differences were observed between the symbolic behavior, both verbal and nonverbal, of the men and women patients. The women tended to adhere to the etiquette of language and be more formal in appearance than were the men. This contrast was more noticeable in the coed sessions, where the men ended up preempting much of the lecture time. The women also exhibited much care in their personal appearance (Wilsnack, 1973), although the men were also neatly dressed. Several women remarked on different occasions that while "on booze," they didn't care what they "looked like." In addition, the women rarely used "four-letter" words, whether in coed or segregated sessions. Similarly, their voices, laughter, and anger were all restrained. They did not cry in these sessions. Even the younger women displayed "ladylike" posture. In fact, quite a few women expressed an open concern over being ladylike. For example, one stated that she vowed to learn to drink like a lady. Another claimed that while drunk she was so unladylike that her language would have made men blush. One patient stated that she was told not to use "them" (obscene language) when young and would rather not use them. She seemed provoked when such disapproved language was occasionally used by one of the other women. The women referred to each other as "girls" while the staff and the male patients referred to them as "ladies."

Although the men tried to mind their manners in mixed company, quite a few obscene words were used, particularly in the all-male sessions. Use of these words increased considerably when the counselor was a male. One counselor himself used "s.o.b." and "bastard" in reference to himself as a drunk. Only one, a younger male, used an epithet involving a sexual act and on realizing that the researcher was present, apologized for use of such language. But words like "hell" and "damn" were not uncommon. Another man substantiated a woman patient's claim about the language of the drunken person, stating that when drunk he used "foul language" that shouldn't be used in "mixed company." It is quite possible that the men seemed more comfortable in the presence of male counselors, in part because they did not have to guard their language and manners. References and innuendos regarding women and sex occurred several times.

In contrast, there was only one reference to sex among the women, and this only in an indirect manner. A patient asked if her boredom at x-rated movies was typical women's reaction since her husband seemed to enjoy them. All of the women expressed their agreement with her feelings. But this incident was brief. The women did not seem to resent the institution's rule forbidding "fraternization," while the men complained about it. The women, unlike the men, did not seem any more comfortable in the company of a counselor of their own sex than one of the opposite sex. They definitely exhibited a preferential liking for a particular, younger male counselor. They joked about his good looks and called a patient "lucky" when this male counselor chose to sit beside her. But he seemed mostly to evoke comparison with their own sons and perhaps it was this identification that made them feel more at home with him.

The male and female patients differed in the extent to which they were frank and open in group sessions. Although the younger women were somewhat more open, the males in general were less reticent in speaking about the facility, confinement, and treatment. The frankest statement on the part of the women occurred when one remarked that all she wanted to do was get high. Another started with the preamble "I hate to say this here . . . ," and claimed that if she didn't have children and a husband and was not involved in the community as a family, she wouldn't care what she did. However, the male alcoholics were much more forthright. One remarked, when the group had to move to a room other than the one in which the sessions were originally held because the windows were being sealed, that he supposed that "they" (the staff) didn't want the patients to get high smelling the glue. The group continued along this vein for a while. On another occasion, the same patient demanded with some anger in his voice, to know why the staff wouldn't allow him the use of a mouthrinse. A second male complained that he had been in the facility for several days without yet having met with his counselor. And several patients complained that it was expensive to stay in the facility. Indeed, one man stated that the cost of stay was his reason for leaving early against the staff's wishes, although the staff claimed that was a rationalization since he was apparently successful.

While the monetary aspect of the stay was expressed as being important to the men, only two women made any reference to the financial aspect of their treatment. An older, nonworking, divorced woman expressed concern that she might not be able to afford the extended stay the staff recommended. Another stated that as long as her estranged husband was willing to pay, she would stay the recommended period. Being breadwinners, the men were perhaps more concerned with meeting their financial obligations and getting their money's worth. But even those whose insurance or employer was paying for the treatment conveyed the belief that it was all in return for their labor.

The male patients' criticisms centered also on the facility's food. It is only natural that, while in confinement without much else to do, food takes on a special significance. Almost all agreed that the food at the facility was terrible. They complained that although they were supposed to choose ahead of time what they preferred from the menu, they were never served what they wanted and ordered. One man declared that his meat was "green" and went on to elaborate in graphic detail what it resembled. Quite a bit of time was spent on discussing food and the cost of the facility. The women seemed least concerned with this aspect of their stay.

Although both men and women were discontented about their confinement and limited physical activities, the men were more vocal about it. The women mildly remarked that their brains were getting "pickled" or they complained about the small room in which the sessions were held occasionally. The men openly expressed their delight at the administrative decision to increase their "walk time" from one half hour to one hour. This blunt approach of the men continued regarding some of the treatment tactics and strategies.

Several of the men demanded that an AA sponsored movie, "If You Love Me," not be shown to their families since they objected to the portrayal of the male alcoholic in that movie. Although the women concurred that it was "heavy," they did not vocalize their objections, if any. Apparently either the women failed to identify with the male protagonist or felt powerless to demand that it not be shown to their families.

The men were also quite vocal in expressing their criticism of and objection to some of the AA volunteers who were an integral part of the lecture and "bridge" sessions. Perhaps this was because they resisted accepting the label "alcoholic" and the disease concept on which AA ideology is based. Several of the men commented that there were a few "AA types" who went after the patients like "barracuda smelling blood." One remarked that "they" like putting people on the (proverbial) "hot seat." These men openly questioned the lack of professional qualifications of the AA volunteers to administer psychotherapy-like treatment, which they claimed "went too far" at times. Someone said that these volunteers did not know when to stop. On the other hand, several mentioned on different occasions that frequent and regular attendance at AA seems to help them remain sober.

The men were not afraid to express their skepticism of the view of alcoholism as a disease and of various aspects of AA, and resisted participating in labeling themselves "alcoholics." One man was quite antagonistic and made negative comments about AA's style, beliefs, and religious fervor. He stated that "they" were substituting booze with "born again" religion. Another poked fun at the revivalist tone of an AA tape during a lecture session; while one man remarked that even after regular attendance, AA meetings failed to help put together some "loose ends."

In contrast, the women were quite accepting of AA and the disease concept. For example, one woman mentioned how afraid she was for her son and daughter-in-law (both drinkers), since "it may run in the family." "Catch it before it happens" was her wish for their well-being. Two other women referred respectively to their spouse and mother not understanding their disease. And several seemed to believe that alcoholism was some kind of a biological, allergic condition. In addition, these women seemed to subscribe to the notion of alcoholism as a "family disease." This belief did not quite clearly come across in the men's sessions. The women tended to draw parallels between their alcoholism and other ailments. One remarked while discussing another's proposed trip abroad after "graduation": "If you had a heart attack and the doctor told you not to go, would you?" This same woman declared that she decided to grow out of drugs since booze was legal. She claimed she has now "accepted" that she is an alcoholic and she has to live with that disease.

The men were not afraid of bluntly expressing their evaluations of peers directly. For example, there were no preambles, qualifiers, or euphemisms while critiquing one another. When the group was solicited for its reaction to one man's decision to leave against the wishes of the staff, the men openly conveyed their belief that they did not buy the rationalization he used to justify his decision. This was, in fact, the hottest issue ever to be discussed in the men's group during the period of observation. Similarly, the men were critical of another man's tendency to "intellectualize." But all these comments and criticisms were tempered by a sense of detachment. There was no attempt to change the point of view of the person of whose behavior they disapproved.

The women, on the other hand, were not quite as forthright or dispassionate in conveying their opinions of their peers. Their critique almost always tended to be observations of the positive qualities of the peer being evaluated. For example, one woman was complimented as a very "together person," while the session was supposed to focus on her "character defects" that may cause her to "slip." If and when there was any criticism at all, they prefaced it with assurances of their love, understanding, and concern as well as support for the person being evaluated. Among the women, there was also a tendency to digress and deflect. For example, two women started with assurances to another that they do understand how she felt "really . . . !" The women evidently were not accustomed to saying what they precisely felt, perhaps reflecting their sensitivity to other people's feelings. This lack of candor on the part of women was apparent in several other incidents. When, for example, I asked why a particular female patient was absent, one woman claimed that she did not know, although evidently all knew that the absent woman was down with an allergy. Later in the research, the same reluctant patient was the first to confide to me that she had heard that a younger patient was pregnant. This seeming paranoia on the part of women culminated in a counselor's confrontation with one woman when he asked her if she felt she couldn't tell the truth at the facility.

Although reluctant to discuss peers, the women were concerned with the idea of "sharing with the group"—that is, trusting the peers and counselors in the group sessions. A newly admitted patient's distrust of the nonfamilial environment seemed to have upset some of the women who repeatedly assured her that she can trust the "group." When one woman decided to leave treatment and her spouse to "head south," but refused to discuss the prospects of it, they pointedly remarked about her lack of trust in them. Similarly, when a rather withdrawn young woman refused to participate, the women assured her that she was in the right place to start developing trust in others. The women also tended to yield readily to peer pressure. Many decisions and plans for the future seemed to have been (at least temporarily) shelved because of the persuasion of the peers and counselors.

Level of Affectivity Exhibited

Unlike the men who seemed more detached, the women patients were clearly more demonstrative of their affections and feelings for each other. When one woman was discharged, the others congregated around the "graduate" kissing, hugging, and crying. In fact, when one young woman upon arrival spent much time crying and claiming that she missed her family and hugging her mother, all the older women tried to console her by saying that although they were not quite her mother, they would hug her a lot and that she could hug them anytime she wanted. Another woman was suffering with an allergy and all went to visit her and, in her words, "held my hands."

The expressive role orientation of the women was conveyed in yet other ways. One woman did not hesitate to cry while recollecting how drunk she was when her daughter needed her during a difficult childbirth. Another started crying when she admitted to bottling up all her emotions, including her love for her son, for too long. On another occasion, one woman broke down in tears at the prospect of losing her husband. Another cried about her fear of her husband's harassment if she were to leave him but continue to live in the same state, contending that the resultant tensions may threaten her sobriety. A homesick new resident cried for two continuous days claiming that she felt deserted by her family and felt imprisoned. She broke down completely when narrating how important talking to her psychiatrist was for her while the rules of the facility restricted telephoning anyone. Chokingly, she stated that he couldn't possibly feed her "booze through the telephone." It was not uncommon for the women to go looking for tissues, and one of their standby jokes was about keeping the kleenex company in business.

Envy and jealousy sprung up readily among the women. In one instance, this occurred when a peer preempted several sessions to discuss "her" unique problem. One woman declared loudly that her reason for not attending one of the earlier sessions was that she was "tired of listening to _____'s problems." The women competed not only for the attention of the staff, the male patients, and their peers, but also to demonstrate how much more loved and, therefore, superior they were as mothers and spouses. The upstaging reported below is a case in point. One woman circulated a picture of her teenage daughter and dog; this was followed by another showing off the pictures of her two young children. A third started reading passages from her daughter's letter. Several of the other women then had to refer to the loving and lovely letters and dialogues with their families. The men, however, exhibited some envy and competition toward their wealthier peers' better jobs, intellectual sophistication, and articulateness.

Jealousies regarding other issues also emerged among the women. For example, the youngest of the female patients was allowed (as an exception) to make two phone calls within the first week of her admission since she was refusing to cooperate unless she was allowed to make the phone calls. This led to such an uproar that it was the focus of attention and reference in several group and staff meetings. There were complaints about such partiality and grumblings about differential enforcement of institutional rules. A great deal of anger was expressed against a woman patient who got away with her refusal to participate in the sessions by lying in her bed. Another was allowed to jog within the premises and several of the women complained that she was allowed many concessions while they weren't; they wanted more walks, outings, and movement. The staff referred to such incidents of discontent as "the troops are restless."

Yet another aspect of the women's expressive role orientation was indicated by the manner in which dyadic and other friendship formations and cliques emerged among them. Affinities, loyalties, and admirations within such groups were also openly expressed. The male patients did not engage in such conduct.

SUMMARY AND IMPLICATIONS

It would be unwarranted to generalize beyond the findings of limited participant observation of a small group of men and women in one setting. But to the extent that the patients observed in this facility resemble alcoholics generally, the different behaviors, orientations, and concerns revealed by them in group sessions might have some implications for treatment strategy.

Among the differences observed in this research, several appear to be related to therapy:

1. The women were blatantly reluctant to take the initiative in communicating the issues that concerned them while the men were much more aggressive in this regard.
2. While the women were concerned with expressing their anger and frustration at all, the men were concerned with expressing such feeling in an appropriate manner.
3. The women were more willing to exhibit their emotions by crying but the men seemed detached even about their most intimate concerns.
4. The male alcoholic patients were clearly interested in the mechanics of remaining sober, treating the prospect as a practical problem to be resolved. Women, in contrast, seemed more concerned with what others would think of them for being an alcoholic and in treatment.
5. The men exhibited concern over how to deal with their general occupational and, to some extent, interpersonal roles while the women focused on specific behaviors of the significant others in their lives.
6. While the female alcoholics were timid about making issues, the male alcoholic patients engaged in confrontations without much concern.
7. The women were concerned with outward physical appearance and demeanor while the men were not.

One of the rationales behind the extended period of therapy beyond mere detoxification is that once an alcoholic has "dried out" the crises of the pharmacological effects of alcohol, the new environment free of family and other demands under the guidance of trained and empathetic treatment personnel will be conducive to their learning skills to identify those habits, behaviors and situations that propel them toward abusing alcohol and the ways of coping with these and the demands of living. Presumably, alcoholics equipped with such knowledge and information on the effects of alcohol and other chemicals on the body, and their psychosocial impact on the individual, will be able to maintain sobriety. In addition, the establishment of a supportive network consisting of understanding professionals, peers, family, friends and work associates will help alcoholics beyond their therapeutic-community experience.

We know very little about the impact of therapy on the prognosis of alcoholic men and women regarding the following issues: (1) the gender of the counselor; (2) the type of technique used (e.g., individual vs. group therapy); (3) the type of counselor used (e.g., recovering alcoholic vs. one who has had no drinking related problem, counselors with personal experience with alcoholism vs. those who have been exposed to alcoholism specific therapeutic training); (4) therapy sessions and facilities which are segregated by (both counselor and patient) gender; (5) therapy that is oriented to confirming traditional gender roles vs. consciousness raising sessions. These variables may help us tailor the treatment techniques to suit the needs of the patients.

Given the limited resources available for any curative effort and the need to allocate resources to the most effective treatment strategies and techniques, we need some rational bases for advocating certain treatment practices. Remedial techniques chosen on an ad hoc basis are not too far from the arbitrary rationale of folk medicine men.

REFERENCES

Bales, Robert F. "A Set of Categories for the Analysis of Small Group Interaction," *American Sociological Review,* 15 (April, 1950):257-263.

Bateman, N. I. and D. M. Peterson "Factors Related to Outcome of Treatment for Hospitalized White Male and Female Alcoholics," *Journal of Drug Issues,* 2 (1972):66-74.

Beckman, Linda J. "Women Alcoholics: A Review of Social and Psychological Studies," *Journal of Studies on Alcohol,* 36 (1975):797-824.

Blume, Sheila B. "Group Psychotherapy in the Treatment of Alcoholics," in Sheldon Zimberg, John Wallace, and Sheila B. Blume (eds.) *Practical Approaches to Alcoholism Psychotherapy* (New York: Plenum, 1978):63-76.

Curlee, Joan "Alcoholic Women: Some Considerations for Further Research," *Bulletin of the Menninger Clinic,* 31 (1967):154-163.

_____ "Women Alcoholics," *Federal Probation,* 32 #1 (1968):16-20.

_____ "A Comparison of Male and Female Patients at an Alcoholism Treatment Center," *Journal of Psychology,* 74 (1970):239-247.

_____ "Sex Differences in Patient Attitudes Toward Alcoholism Treatment," *Quarterly Journal of Studies on Alcohol,* 32 (1971):643-650.

Duberman, Lucile *Marriage and Other Alternatives,* 2ed. (New York: Praeger, 1977).

Kinsey, Barry A. *The Female Alcoholic: A Social Psychological Study* (Springfield, Ill.: Thomas, 1966).

Lisansky, Edith S. "Alcoholism in Women: Social and Psychological Concomitants. I. Social History Data," *Quarterly Journal of Studies on Alcohol* 15 (1957):588-623.

Pemberton, D. A. "A Comparison of the Outcome of Treatment in Female and Male Alcoholics," *British Journal of Psychiatry,* 113 (1967):367-373.

Rimmer, J., F. N. Pitts, Jr., and T. Reich "Alcoholism. II. Sex, Socioeconomic Status and Race in Two Hospitalized Samples," *Quarterly Journal of Studies on Alcohol,* 32 (1971): 942-952.

Saunders, Bill "Psychological Aspects of Women and Alcohol," in *Women and Alcohol* (London: Tavistock, 1980):67-100.

Schuckit, M. A. and Elizabeth R. Morissey "Alcoholism in Women: Some Clinical and Social Perspectives With an Emphasis on Possible Subtypes," in Milton Greenblatt and Marc A. Schuckit (eds.) *Alcoholism Problems in Women and Children* (New York: Grune and Stratton, 1976):5-35.

Tamerin, John S., A. Tolor and B. Harrington "Sex Differences in Alcoholics' Self and Spouse Perceptions," *The American Journal of Drug and Alcohol Abuse,* 3 (1978):457-472.

Tamerin, John S. "The Psychotherapy of Alcoholic Women," in Sheldon Zimberg, John Wallace and Sheila Blume (eds.) *Practical Approaches to Alcoholism Psychotherapy* (New York: Plenum, 1978):183-203.

Wilsnack, Sharon C. "Sex Role Identity in Female Alcoholism," *Journal of Abnormal Psychology,* 82 (1973):253-261.

_____ "The Impact of Sex Roles on Women's Alcohol Use and Abuse," in Milton Greenblatt and Marc A. Schuckit (eds.) *Alcoholism Problems in Women and Children* (New York: Grune and Stratton, 1976):37-63.

Conclusion:
On the Horns of Three Dilemmas
in Alcoholism Treatment:
Propriety, Professionalism and Power

Merton M. Hyman
David L. Strug
S. Priyadarsini

In reading the 10 papers we saw several repetitive themes which gave us a gratifying sense of order and structure in the field of alcoholism treatment. These themes emerge from the authors' substantive discussion, not from any theoretical positions. However, the authors whose papers revolve around the issues of differential power between alcoholics and treatment, custodial and administrative personnel clearly indicate an awareness of broader issues raised by their papers.

PROPRIETY

A basic theme in Dr. Lender's paper is that the special stigma visited upon women alcoholics has caused women alcoholics to avoid or delay entry into alcoholism treatment programs; hence on the whole, they were in the past, and are even today, more advanced in their alcoholism, and worse in physical health than men alcoholics first coming into treatment. As the author points out, the attitudes regarding alcoholism among women versus men are part of a larger pattern of more severe demands regarding propriety made by society on women than on men. These impediments to women alcoholics seeking help stem from feelings and attitudes of others in their social network as well as themselves and continue, if somewhat abated, even at present. Beckman and Amaro (1982) found that women alcoholics had less support than did men alcoholics from significant others in seeking help for their alcohol problems. Worse yet, they found that women alcoholics often encountered opposition from their relatives and friends in seeking help for their alcoholism, which was rarely encountered by men alcoholics.

Dr. Priyadarsini's study of women and men in group therapy reveals the overwhelming burden of inhibitions on women in therapy, especially in groups and above all when men are present, in discussing their problems, especially anger and resentment toward others. This, too, is part of a larger pattern of differing societal definitions of what is appropriate behavior in women vs. men. Such differentiation can impede the process of women alcoholics toward recovery.

An important issue, not raised by either Drs. Priyadarsini or Lender, needs to be elucidated. That is that the very discrimination against women regarding definitions of appropriate behavior is partly responsible for the lower prevalence of problem-drinking and other problematic behavior among them.

Traditionally the upbringing of and the expectations for women have been oriented toward preparing them for adult roles in which their lives were to be far more circumscribed than those of men. No doubt these different upbringings and expectations played an important role in causing women to be, on the whole, less risk-taking than men (except with regard to childbirth). It is probable that if high-risk drinking behavior and risk-taking in general were regarded as no more improper behavior for women than for men the prevalence of problem drinking and problematic behavior in general would have been far greater among women than they actually were. (Greater equality between the sexes, such as has been evolving during the past century, and is still evolving, has been and will continue to be a mixed blessing.)

We are faced with a fundamental dilemma that a more even-handed definition of propriety for men and women, essential for inducing women alcoholics not to avoid or delay their entry into treatment, might well raise the prevalence of alcoholism and alcohol misuse among women closer to the levels found among men.[1]

PROFESSIONALISM

The description of the student body of the Rutgers Center of Alcohol Studies (CAS) Summer School of Alcohol Studies (SSAS) by Dr. Milgram mirrors the radical changes in composition of alcoholism treatment personnel over the last 40 years.

When the SSAS began in 1943, most of the students were in professions that brought them into some contact with alcoholics (teachers and administrators; ministers and other religious workers; welfare workers; and law enforcement officers). Alcoholism treatment was not yet a separate profession, alcohol studies were not yet a separate discipline and alcoholics or problem drinkers were only some of the people that these professions dealt with. Forty years later well over half of the students of the SSAS were alcoholism counselors, members of a distinct profession and trained in a distinct discipline.

The evolution of alcoholism treatment as a modern profession and discipline is also discussed in Mr. Keller's paper. The early attempts at behavioral conditioning to lead alcoholics to abstinence (e.g., putting worms or insects into alcohol beverages; no doubt producing some successes, as most folk remedies do) seems to us primitive indeed. The early attempts to treat alcoholics through psychotherapy were based on religious rather than psychological views of behavior. However, some of these were, no doubt, sometimes successful.

Yet another indication of the growth of alcoholism treatment as a modern profession and discipline, as depicted by Mr. Keller, is the sheer variety of different types of alcoholism treatment offered at the same institutions and agencies. However, this probably reflects an intermediate, not an advanced, state of alcoholism treatment effectiveness. If alcoholism treatment were on a solid scientific footing and with higher rates of effectiveness, there would probably be a decrease in variety of treatment modalities.[2]

Why is professionalism in the area of alcoholism treatment a problem? This "problem" of professionalism lies in the complex web of interaction—specialization of developing bureaucracies, public sector employment (directly or indirectly via third-party payments), a clientele primarily of those with low levels of social and economic resources, and uninformed fickleness of the public as to salient social and other problems.

Specialization of alcoholism treatment as a separate profession and discipline makes it difficult for alcoholism treatment personnel to change their profession and find new employment in other fields. Alcoholism treatment personnel have a stake in maintaining the status quo, which can easily take precedence over ministering to the needs of extant or potential clients or patients. Their positions usually are in some bureaucracy; hence their vested interest (for their self-esteem as well as financial security) rests not only in the contin-

uance of their own position but in the continuance of the bureaucratic apparatus in which they function.

This itself might not pose a problem. But alcoholism (and drug)
treatment, research, education and treatment-training personnel
have a problem in maintaining their positions not faced by other
public sector personnel.

Most alcoholism treatment personnel work either in agencies and
institutions that are themselves part of government apparatuses or
receive funding from government units. (Many private alcoholism
treatment agencies and institutions also receive government support.
Furthermore, treatment facilities paid for by private insurance companies can also be considered, broadly interpreted, as part of the
"public sector." Indirectly the public pay for these.) As Dr. Blume
has pointed out, most clients or patients of alcoholism treatment programs have low resources at intake. Some of the low prestige rubs
off on the treatment personnel. However, this has been gradually
changing; and people who follow such careers are being more accepted as respected professionals.

Greater acceptance by other professions and by the public of
alcoholism (and drug misuse) treatment, education, research and
treatment-training as legitimate professions does not solve a basic
problem confronting these professionals: fickleness of the public,
expressed via governmental agencies, as to what are salient social
problems, worthy of public funds' being allocated to cope with
them.

The very frequent changes in course material at the Summer
School of Alcohol Studies and of other educational programs offered by the Center of Alcohol Studies (CAS), as set forth by Dr.
Milgram, clearly reflect the fickleness of interest in and the funding
of different types of alcoholism treatment, education, research and
treatment-training programs. This is not the fault of the CAS.
Rather the CAS, to continue its existence, must be sensitive to
changes in demand for different courses and programs. We find it
difficult to believe that these numerous changes reflect rapidly
changing objective societal needs. Rather, we believe, they reflect
the faddishness of general or of influential public opinion. Funding
largely depends on what issues or goals happen to be salient, to
"grab" the public in a given point of time.

The manipulating and maneuvering of people in the fields of
alcoholism treatment, education, research and treatment-training as
described by Wiener (1981) can be readily attributed to the insecuri-

ty of personnel in these fields rather than to any special penchant for these activities by people in those professions.

Besides fickleness of the public (or segments thereof) there are reasons to believe that discussions as to how much funds to allocate to different types of facilities are determined by past and present general or influential public opinion which is, on the whole, uninformed, rather than based on objective needs.

One example in the alcohol/drug field is as follows: comparing results of a general household survey of alcohol and drug use and misuse with a census of treatment facility capacities in Pennsylvania, Glasser and Greenberg (1975) found that the ratio of alcohol misusers to treatment capacity was 10 times as great as the ratio of drug misusers to treatment capacity.[3]

This aspect of the uninformed nature of general or influential public opinion with regard to the need for public facilities of different types is by no means confined to the coping with alcohol and drug misuse problems. A very gross example of a different type can be seen in regional and state comparisons of inmates of psychiatric hospitals and of jails and prisons (the two chief institutions in the U.S. through which the public copes with deviance among adults).

On the whole, the Northeastern states have many more people in mental hospitals than in jails/prisons and the Southwestern states have many more people in jails/prisons than in psychiatric hospitals. In 1969, prior to the deinstitutionalization movement for psychiatric patients, New York had about three times as many people in mental hospitals as in jails/prisons and California had over twice as many people in jails/prisons as in mental hospitals (U.S. Bureau of the Census, 1976). New York had a ratio of people in psychiatric hospitals to those in jails/prisons more than six times as great as had California.[4]

It strains the imagination to posit that in 1969 there were three times as many mentally ill people as criminals in New York and twice as many criminals as mentally ill people in California. Rather, these figures suggest that our society has two methods of trying to cope with deviance—prisons and mental hospitals—and the past and current public opinion as to how to cope with deviant behavior, not objective needs for different types of facilities, determine the number and capacities of these facilities.

It is not surprising, therefore, that people whose specialized careers have focused on treatment of (and ancilliary functions such as research on and education about) troubled people and who are overwhelmingly dependent for their financial security and career self-images on the largesse of the public (or segments thereof) with its whims, fads and uninformed ideas, should be concerned with the maintenance of their positions and of the bureaucracies which sustain them.

At times these concerns can take precedence over the duties that the "healers" owe either to their patients or clients or to the general public.

As alcoholism treatment personnel are the link between the public (via their governments at various levels) and the alcoholic patients or clients they are supposed to help, this leads us to the third dilemma of alcoholism treatment: use and misuse of power.

POWER

As with the dilemmas of propriety and professionalism, the dilemma of power, its use and misuse is not a one-sided problem.

A certain leverage over alcoholics has been found to be important in helping them to recover. Part of the ideology of Al-Anon is that the relatives and friends of alcoholics should not be too protective in shielding the alcoholic from such unfortunate events as arrest and loss of employment—such confronting experience can galvanize some alcoholics into squarely facing their problem and try to do something about it.

Personnel of companies which have alcoholism treatment programs have found that usually only the threat of losing their jobs influence alcoholic employees to use alcoholism rehabilitation (ALC-REHAB) programs (Heyman, 1978; Trice and Roman, 1972).

Hyman (1985) conducted a follow-up, 14-16 years after intake at an out-patient ALC-REHAB clinic. Not surprisingly, stays at ALC-REHAB hospitals prior to intake are associated with favorable outcomes. However, serious and/or repeated troubles with the law and stays at psychiatric hospitals (for other than ALC-REHAB) prior to intake and social intercession by the clinic on behalf of clients with agents of external authority (e.g., courts, employers, welfare agencies) were also associated with favorable outcomes. A combination of prior stays at ALC-REHAB hospitals with two or three of the other interventions mentioned above were very strongly predictive of favorable outcomes among those with low economic resources (no regular work and/or living in poverty during most of the two years before intake). All these experiences provide leverages whereby the community can pressure alcoholics to start on the road to recovery.[5]

Dr. Rodin et al. have well described the problems that have emerged from the attempt during the 1970s to replace coercive with therapeutic methods in coping with chronic public intoxication. First, as soon as public inebriates are detoxified there is little that can be done directly to propel them into treatment (in the REHAB sense; after a fashion DETOX is also "treatment"). After all, under the new laws they have not committed a legal offense, and they cannot be "sentenced" to "therapy" as they could previously be sentenced to the county workhouse. Most DETOX patients, especially recidivists, do not enter REHAB programs, a phenomenon also reported by other researchers cited by the authors, and by Richman and Smart (1981).

Second, the low levels of social resources of patients (at intake) are associated with poor prognosis. We might add that this is also found for REHAB patients (for systematic arrays or collations of dozens of studies, see Costello, 1980; and Gibbs and Flanagan, 1977). It is probably even more so for DETOX-only patients.

Third, the "revolving door" in and out of jails (as first phrased by Pittman, 1958 and subsequently reported by many others) has become a "spinning door" in and out of DETOX centers (to use Room's phrase).

Fourth, just as skid row alcoholics had, in earlier decades, learned to "use the system" of jails, mental hospitals and missions so they have learned to "use the system" of DETOX centers, a phenomenon also noted by other researchers.

From the descriptions by Rodin et al. it appears that the relations between DETOX personnel and DETOX patients is a cat and mouse game. The help providers are the cats who try to lure the skid row alcoholics into REHAB programs and, theoretically, into recovery. The skid row alcoholics are the mice who try to grab some cheese (DETOX and some immediate material help such as food and lodging) without being forced to give up their way of life.

A unique study depicting the humane latent functions of what is technically a coercive bureaucratic institution, the county workhouse, is presented by Dr. Andrews. She found that customary arrangements between "regulars" (habitual, recidivist alcoholic inmates) and guards were mutually congenial.

Inmates typically spend about half of the year in the workhouse, with sentences for public drunkenness and similar offenses usually ranging from 30 to 90 days. Within the limits of their lay knowledge, guards handled acute intoxication and withdrawal symptoms remarkably well and were concerned with inmate well-being. Nutritious food, clean and warm shelter, protection from violence and about six hours a day of moderate outdoor manual work raising produce and poultry resulted in inmates being physically fit by the time they completed their sentences. Inmates also developed some self-esteem, becoming experts at various aspects of farming, repair work, etc.

The overt function of the workhouse is to relieve the public of the "nuisance" of public inebriation. Its latent function is that of protecting the health and increasing the life-expectancy of chronic public inebriates and provide useful work for them to do. The humane nature of this institution is all the more remarkable in that it is an inherently coercive one, far from being a "country club." If, as a result of some well intentioned "liberal" motives, sentences had been halved, those alcoholics would probably have died or become deteriorated much earlier.

Probably not many jails and workhouses are as humane as the one described above. However, the observations of Dr. Andrews over a period of two years provide clear proof that a humane correctional facility is much superior to DETOX shelters with their rapidly revolving doors in protecting the lives and health of (usually homeless) chronic public inebriates. The public need have no guilt feelings that such institutions also reduce the nuisance of public intoxication. The benefits to the inmates are even greater.

Dr. Andrews has pointed out that most of the workhouse inmates do not want "treatment." For them, being forced by law to undergo "therapy" would actually be a greater interference with their liberty than being sentenced to the workhouse.

To present a balanced picture, it is necessary to discuss the misuse of power. The most obvious example would be sentencing public inebriates to excessively lengthy terms in jails and workhouses. This does not appear to have happened with regard to the workhouse described by Dr. Andrews. However, even in that humane institution there was some abuse of power by the staff; a former inmate who was an expert at, say, raising turkeys might be brought from the streets back to the workhouse if there were an unexpected need for his services!

Changes in law and public opinion during the 1970s as how to cope with public intoxication have greatly reduced misuse of power via excessive or unfair sentences. Rather, the greatest potentiality of misuse of power is in the ability of those who are charged with helping alcoholics to deny them desperately needed food, shelter and medical care which can be provided by and provisions for future social services which can be arranged by staffs of in-house residences (e.g., half-way houses, DETOX facilities). This potential misuse of power applies not only to chronic public inebriates but to any alcoholics who have few or no social and economic resources on which they can rely.[6]

The most flagrant misuse of power discussed in these papers is the case of the tyrannical cook in the half-way house for women described by Drs. Volpe and Rooney. Since residence in that institution was voluntary there were no legal barriers to residents leaving if they were dissatisfied with the way the house was being run. But most of the residents were unemployed, penniless and with little, if any, support from relatives and friends. They needed the half-way house until they could get on their feet, just to survive.

It is important to note that the tyrannical cook could not have interfered with the running of the house and disrupted treatment without at least tacit support from the director, whose opinions on treatment and recovery were similar to those of the cook on whom he relied for information (usually given behind the manager's back) on goings-on at the house.

It is possible that, however unsatisfactory the views of the director (and the cook) were regarding the uselessness of professional psychological help (in contrast to AA), the problems in this house would not have been so severe if the managers had had the same views as the director. Although directors could maneuver to fire the managers, the actual hiring and firing was done by a corporation. Hence there was a succession of managers (seven in three years), itself a disrupting force. The key problem, then, appears to have been intrastaff conflicts, to the detriment of residents' welfare.

Somewhat less gross than the situation described by Volpe and Rooney in the half-way house for women, but nevertheless potentially harmful to the patients' well-being, is the situation in the Alcoholism Treatment Unit of a Psychiatric Hospital described by Dr. Tremper. In that institution, psychiatric social workers (the lowest level of professionals there) were often callous to patients' needs, restricted their freedom to a greater extent than was necessary and thus created a situation which forced patients to be more dependent on the staff for even minor help (e.g., making a phone call) than is necessary for treatment. To salve their consciences the staff defined patients' requests as due to the excessive "dependency" (largely created by the staff itself) and questioned the "motivation" of patients to recover.

Like women in the half-way house described above, men in the Alcoholism Treatment Unit had, on the whole, low levels of social and economic resources. Most of them were in need of "time out" from drinking and a chance to build up their physical health; many also needed social services after their six-week stay. Hence they were at the mercy of the staff.

There were several sources of frustration facing the staff who had the most contact with patients, the psychiatric social workers, who were lowest on the professional "pecking order."

First, low levels of social and economic resources of most patients at intake resulted in low prestige being accorded to the staff members who had the greatest amount of contact with the patients by the personnel of higher echelons in the bureaucracy.[7]

Second, prognosis is, on the whole, poor for alcoholics who have low levels of social and economic resources at intake (even among REHAB patients or clients; Costello, 1980, Gibbs and Flanagan, 1977). And, in fact, through frequent actual or sought-for readmission and thorough feedback from other agencies of former patients resuming their drinking, the staff was fully aware of their low "success" rate.

Third, and perhaps most important, the social workers were simultaneously subject to three, often conflicting, pressures. These were: (1) patients and their relatives, (2) administrations of the state psychiatric hospital complex (itself part of the state department of institutions and agencies) of which the alcoholism unit is part, and (3) the State Division of Alcoholism Control, itself under the jurisdiction of and partly funded by the State Department of Health.

On the one hand, the staff of the unit had to respond to the administrative needs of the psychiatric hospital of which it was a part. On the other hand, the unit, being at that time the only state inpatient ALC-REHAB facility, was expected to accept referrals from numerous sources. Other agencies and outpatient counselors tried to use the unit as a "dumping ground" to send clients who had no place to live. Unit staff were urged to attend statewide meetings of the Division of Alcoholic Control and to work closely with outpatient counselors on mutual clients. Realistically, demands from two lines of authority could not possibly be satisfied with the very limited resources of the unit.

Small wonder, then, that patients, by far the least powerful of the three demanding parties, were given short shrift.

Professionalism in alcoholism treatment, itself a worthy goal, aggravated some of the problems faced by the least powerful of the staff, the social workers. Specializing in the treatment of alcoholics, and dependent on the public sector for employment, it was not easy for them to find new employment. They would have to be saints not to give much greater priority to the demands of their superiors (two separate lines of bureaucratic authority at that) than to the needs of their patients.

Another problematic aspect of the use and misuse of power is that of control over readmissions. Theoretically, the Alcoholism Treatment Unit described by Dr. Tremper and the DETOX centers described by Rodin et al. and by Rubington are not supposed to turn away any alcoholic in need of the services of those facilities. In practice, though, first-time admissions are provided to all of those who are in need and who request the services of the DETOX centers (and most of those in need of the services of the [REHAB] Alcoholism Treatment Unit), the staffs of these facilities exercise considerable control over readmissions.

Technically, the staffs of these facilities are violating the law. Practically, however, the resources of these facilities are much too limited to admit all those in need of and who seek admission. In controlling readmissions the staff are trying to provide a maximum of services to alcoholics within the limited means at their disposal. Given the limited number of openings available, it seems to us as well as to others in the field that giving openings to alcoholics without any or with only a few previous admissions is a better way of using limited resources than giving these openings to alcoholics with known poor "track records" who have entered and exited the "revolving" (or rather "spinning") doors again and again.

SUMMARY

Three dilemmas in alcoholism treatment have been discussed:

1. The removal of the stigma of alcoholism from women to encourage early entry into treatment might well actually result in an increase of high-risk drinking, and consequently of alcoholism

among women (or any other group on whom there have been traditionally strong sanctions against heavy drinking and drunkenness [such as Jews]).

2. Professionalism, a worthy goal itself, is fraught with dangers in fields such as alcoholism treatment, research and treatment-training. These are specialized fields, overwhelmingly supported (directly or indirectly) by the public sector, and vulnerable to unstable, fickle "moods" of an uninformed public; the saliency of issues for them come and go with little relation to objective situations. This insecurity sometimes results in people in these fields placing their own job security and the continuation of the bureaucracies in which they function above that of the needs of the alcoholics whom they are supposed to help.

3. A certain leverage exercised by the community is very useful in inducing alcoholics to enter REHAB treatment. It is also possible for basically coercive institutions such as workhouses to function in a truly humane way and provide much-needed services for alcoholics.

However, power over alcoholics can be easily misused, to the great detriment of those who need help, by the very people who are supposed to help them recover. The misuse of power, to the detriment of alcoholics in need of help, by those who are supposed to help them is particularly likely to occur when there are intra-staff power struggles or when staff members who have closest contact with patients, clients or residents (usually lowest on the staff totem pole) are themselves subjected to excessive, often conflicting expectations of those above them in the bureaucratic hierarchy.

NOTES

1. It is interesting to note that Johnson (1977, 1978) found that both heavy drinking and problem drinking were more prevalent among women who worked outside the home than among those that didn't and that Corrigan (1980) found that suburban women (mostly housewives) alcoholism patients were more likely to have been criticized for their drinking than had the urban (mostly employed) women alcoholics. Other, not mutually exclusive interpretations can be made.

2. Some therapist-researchers have gone as far as advocating a "cafeteria plan" whereby the therapist and the patient jointly decide what kind of treatment to undertake, with different alternatives discussed prior to treatment (Ewing, 1977; Pattison, 1976; though Pattison did not use that expression). That does not strike us as economical or suitable for people who for years have had great difficulty in managing their lives.

3. Another example from the study of Glasser and Greenberg (1975) is as follows: the ratio of alcohol misusers to treatment capacity was 44 and 55, respectively, in urban and suburban (metropolitan) counties but 255 and 155, respectively, in non-metropolitan counties with small cities and rural counties.

4. In 1980 the differences between New York and California were somewhat smaller. However it is unlikely that changes in objective needs for different types of facilities had been responsible for these changes. For example, in New York State the number of people in federal or state prison facilities decreased 36% from 1960 to 1970 and increased 120% from 1970 to 1981 (my calculations from data on population and inmates, U.S. Bureau of the Census, 1982). Such large changes in one decade could hardly reflect changes in the need for prison facilities even with moderate changes in the demographic composition of the population of New York.

5. There are other, not mutually exclusive, explanations for the findings. First, such experiences make it harder for alcoholics to deny that they are alcoholics. Second, that in having these experiences they meet alcoholics who are much more deteriorated than they are, a healthy reminder of their own possible fates if they continue to drink.

6. Tremper found that some patients in the inpatient REHAB unit he studied were destitute and had nowhere else to go. Strug and Hyman (1981) found that though REHAB inpatients had, on the whole, far richer social networks of close people than DETOX-only patients, there was a minority of REHAB patients with extremely small or no extant networks of close persons from whom they could get any kind of help. Hyman (1985) found that frequent visits (11+) to an outpatient REHAB clinic was mainly motivated by desires for immediate medical help and social services, though clinic personnel perceive their prime function as providing psychological help via counseling and group psychotherapy.

7. This may well be true of other sections of the hospital complex that were not studied intensively by Dr. Tremper.

REFERENCES

Beckman, L. J. and Amaro, H. *Barriers to Treatment Among Anglo Women.* Los Angeles, Alcohol Research Center, Neuropsychiatric Institute University of California, 1982.

Corrigan, E. M. *Alcoholic Women in Treatment.* New York, Oxford University Press, 1980.

Costello, R. M. Alcoholism Treatment Effectiveness: Slicing the Outcome Pie. In: Edwards, S. G. and Grant, M. Eds. *Alcoholism Treatment in Transition.* London, Croom-Helm, 1980.

Ewing, J. A. Matching therapy and patients: The cafeteria plan. *British Journal of Addictions* 72:13-18, 1977. Reprinted in Pattison, E. M. Ed. *Selection of Treatment for Alcoholics.* New Brunswick, N.J. Rutgers Center of Alcohol Studies, 1982.

Gibbs, L. and Flanagan, J. Prognostic indications of alcoholism treatment outcome. *International Journal of Addictions,* 12:1097-1141, 1977.

Glasser, F. B. and Greenberg, S. W. Relationships between treatment facilities and the prevalence of alcoholism and drug abuse. *Journal of Studies on Alcohol,* 36:348-358, 1975.

Heyman, M. M. Alcohol Programs in Industry: The Patients View. (Rutgers Center of Alcohol Studies Monog. No. 12) New Brunswick, N.J., 1978.

Hyman, M. Aging and Alcoholism: A 15-year follow-up. In Gottheil, E., Druley, K. A., Skolada, T. E. and Waxman, H. M., Eds. *The Combined Problems of Alcoholism, Drug Addiction and Aging.* Springfield, Ill., Thomas, 1985.

Johnson, P. B. Sex Differences in Drinking Practices. Report Prepared for the National Institute on Alcohol Abuse and Alcoholism. Santa Monica, Rand Corporation, 1977.

Johnson, P. B. Working Women and Alcohol Use: Preliminary National Data. Paper presented at the meeting of the American Psychological Association, Toronto, Canada, Sept. 1978.

Pattison, E. M. Non-abstinent drinking goals in the treatment of alcoholism: A clinical typology. *Archives of General Psychiatry,* 33:923-930, 1976. Reprinted in Pattison, E. M. Ed. *Selection of Treatment for Alcoholics,* New Brunswick, N.J. Rutgers Center of Alcohol Studies, 1982.

Pittman, D. J. and Gordon, C. W., *Revolving Door,* New Brunswick, N.J. Rutgers Center of Alcohol Studies, 1958.

Richman, A. and Smart, R. G. After how many detoxifications is rehabilitation possible? *Drug and Alcohol Dependency.* 7:233-238, 1981.

Strug, D. L. and Hyman, M. M. Social networks of alcoholics. *Journal of Studies on Alcohol,* 42:855-884, 1981.

Trice, H. M. and Roman, P. M. *Spirits and Demons at Work: Alcoholism and Drugs on the Job.* Ithaca, Cornell University, New York School of Industrial and Labor Relations, 1972.

U. S. Bureau of the Census. *Statistical Abstracts of the United States,* U.S. Government Printing Office, Washington, D.C., Annual.

Weiner, C.L. *The Politics of Alcoholism: Building an Arena Around a Social Problem,* New Brunswick, N.J. Transaction, Inc., 1981.

Index

abstinence, as alcoholism treatment
   goal, 25-26
acupuncture, as alcoholism treatment,
   33-34
Addiction Research Foundation, 12,64
admission
   to detoxification centers, 98-99,111
   refusal of, 105-106
   voluntary nature of, 97,105
affectivity, of female alcoholics, 186,
   192-193
age factors, in detoxification recidivism,
   90
Al-Anon, 7,12,64,202
Alateen, 66
alcohol abuse, alcoholism vs., 23-24
alcohol addiction, alcoholism vs., 24
Alcohol and Drug Problems Association,
   64
alcohol consumption, during Prohibition,
   4
alcohol-dependence syndrome, 24
alcoholic beverages, taxation of, 4
alcoholics, see also chronic public
      inebriates
   attitudes towards Alcoholics
      Anonymous, 190
   authority figure response of, 34
   church ministries for, 7,64
   family of, 202
   female, 41-47
      demographic characteristics of,
         179-180
      emotionality of, 186,192-193
      gender roles of, 43-46,198
      group therapy participation by,
         179-196,198
      in halfway houses, 19-20,161-178
      health status of, 42,51-53,54,197
      "hidden", 41-42,50-51
      historical background of, 42-55

recovery from, 50-51
      sexual promiscuity stereotype of,
         48-49
      significant others' support for,
         197-198
      social stigma of, 9-11,41-57,180,
         197-198,207-208
      solitary drinking by, 41,180
      stereotypes of alcoholics and, 46-50
      temperance movement and, 45-46
      treatment of, 50-51,54,180,197-198
   friends of, 202
   gender-differences of, 179-180, see
      also gender roles
   incarcerated, see also workhouses,
      chronic public inebriates in
      alcoholism treatment for, 36
   institutionalization of, 2,82-83,173-176
   legal status of, 7,97,105,129-130
   public attitudes towards, see also
         social stigma
      historical, 1
      during Prohibition, 71-72
   stereotypes of, 144
      female alcoholics, 47-50
      during nineteenth century, 46-47
Alcoholics Anonymous
   alcoholics' attitudes towards, 190
   in detoxification centers, 119,121,122,
      123,125,126
   founding of, 5,30,60
   halfway house residency and, 163,176
   membership of, 79
      during 1930s, 60
   philosophy of, 5
   religious basis of, 36
   Summer School of Alcohol Studies
      and, 71
alcohol injection, 33
alcoholism
   alcohol abuse vs., 23-24